Rising Serpent: A Guide to Kundalini Awakening

Unlocking Inner Power and Spiritual Transformation

Marcus Mitchell

© Copyright 2024 - All rights reserved.

The content contained within this book may not be reproduced, duplicated or transmitted without direct written permission from the author or the publisher.

Under no circumstances will any blame or legal responsibility be held against the publisher, or author, for any damages, reparation, or monetary loss due to the information contained within this book, either directly or indirectly.

Legal Notice:

This book is copyright protected. It is only for personal use. You cannot amend, distribute, sell, use, quote or paraphrase any part, or the content within this book, without the consent of the author or publisher.

Disclaimer Notice:

Please note the information contained within this document is for educational and entertainment purposes only. All effort has been executed to present accurate, up to date, reliable, complete information. No warranties of any kind are declared or implied. Readers acknowledge that the author is not engaging in the rendering of legal, financial, medical or professional advice. The content within this book has been derived from various sources. Please consult a licensed professional before attempting any techniques outlined in this book.

By reading this document, the reader agrees that under no circumstances is the author responsible for any losses, direct or indirect, that are incurred as a result of the use of information contained within this document, including, but not limited to, errors, omissions, or inaccuracies.

Table of Contents

INTRODUCTION 6

CHAPTER I: Understanding Kundalini Energy 8

Exploring the origins and history of Kundalini 8

The nature of Kundalini energy 11

How Kundalini energy manifests in the body and mind.... 14

CHAPTER II: The Chakra System 19

An in-depth look at the seven chakras 19

Understanding the role of each chakra in Kundalini awakening.. 22

Techniques for balancing and aligning the chakras 26

CHAPTER III: Signs and Symptoms of Kundalini Awakening 31

Recognizing the early signs of Kundalini activation 31

Common physical, emotional, and spiritual symptoms..... 34

Navigating the challenges of Kundalini awakening 37

CHAPTER IV: Preparation for Kundalini Awakening 42

Mind-body practices for preparing the system 42

Cultivating mindfulness and self-awareness 45

Creating a supportive environment for the awakening process 49

CHAPTER V: Kundalini Yoga and Meditation Techniques 53

Introduction to Kundalini yoga 53

Specific yoga poses and meditation techniques for Kundalini awakening.. 56

Breathwork and including visualization exercises 60

CHAPTER VI: The Role of Energy Healing 64

Exploring various energy healing modalities 64

How energy healing can aid in Kundalini activation 67

Working with healers and practitioners 71

CHAPTER VII: Challenges and Solutions 75

Common obstacles faced during Kundalini awakening 75

Strategies for overcoming challenges 78

Seeking guidance and support 82

CHAPTER VIII: Integrating Kundalini Energy into Daily Life 86

Balancing spiritual growth with everyday responsibilities........ 86

Incorporating Kundalini practices into daily routines 89

Nurturing ongoing spiritual development 93

CHAPTER IX: The Spiritual Evolution 97

The profound impact of Kundalini awakening on spiritual evolution... 97

Connecting with higher consciousness 100

Embracing the journey of continuous growth 104

CHAPTER X: Stories of Transformation 108

Real-life accounts of individuals who experienced Kundalini awakening.. 108

Lessons learned, and insights gained 111

Inspiration for those on their own Kundalini journey 114

CHAPTER XI: Beyond Kundalini Awakening 119

Exploring advanced spiritual practices 119

Continuing the journey of self-discovery 123

The limitless potential of a fully awakened Kundalini 128

CONCLUSION 132

INTRODUCTION

In the quiet depths of spiritual exploration, "Rising Serpent" is a guiding light on the transformative path of Kundalini Awakening. This profound book invites seekers and enthusiasts alike to embark on an illuminating journey, delving into the ancient practice of Kundalini and unlocking the inner power that resides within.

As the world seeks deeper connections with the spiritual self, "Rising Serpent" opens a gateway to profound inner realms. This book is not merely a guide; it is a roadmap to understanding and harnessing the potent force of Kundalini, a sacred energy coiled within each individual, waiting to be awakened and harnessed for spiritual evolution.

The introduction unfolds like the awakening of the serpent itself, gradually revealing the essence of Kundalini and its transformative potential. It beckons readers to explore the mystical landscapes of the inner self, where the dormant serpent lies, poised to ascend and unleash spiritual vitality.

"Rising Serpent" introduces the foundational principles of Kundalini Awakening, emphasizing the profound connection between body, mind, and spirit. The narrative weaves through the historical and cultural tapestry of Kundalini practices, offering insights into the diverse methods employed by ancient and contemporary spiritual traditions.

Readers are guided through practices and techniques designed to awaken and balance the Kundalini energy as the pages unfold. "Rising Serpent" is not just a manual but an invitation to set out on a life-changing adventure where the serpentine energy rises, unlocking inner power and initiating a spiritual metamorphosis.

Join us on this immersive exploration, where the ancient wisdom of Kundalini meets the aspirations of the modern seeker. "Rising Serpent" is a companion for those on the path of spiritual awakening, providing insights, guidance, and the keys to unlocking the dormant energy within, fostering a profound spiritual transformation.

CHAPTER I

Understanding Kundalini Energy

Exploring the origins and history of Kundalini

The mystical and spiritual force known as kundalini, thought to remain latent at the base of the spine, has a long history in several ancient societies. This section explores the origins and history of Kundalini, tracing its development through Hinduism and Tantric rituals and its integration into modern spiritual practices. Kundalini's journey is marked by cultural evolution, philosophical interpretations, and the transformative experiences associated with its awakening.

The earliest references to Kundalini can be found in the ancient Hindu scriptures, particularly the Upanishads. These sacred texts describe a coiled serpent, representing dormant divine energy, residing at the base of the spine in the Muladhara Chakra. The concept is closely linked to the broader Hindu belief in the intricate energy system within the human body, known as the Chakra system. Kundalini, in this context, is considered the primal life force that, when awakened, leads to spiritual enlightenment.

The Tantric traditions of ancient India played a pivotal role in shaping and expanding the understanding of Kundalini. Tantra, meaning "loom" or "warp," encompasses a diverse range of spiritual practices aiming to achieve union with the divine. Kundalini is a central element in Tantric philosophy, where it is portrayed as a powerful force capable of transforming the practitioner's consciousness. Tantric texts, such as the "Yoga-Kundalini Upanishad" and the "Hatha Yoga Pradipika," provide detailed instructions on techniques to awaken and channel the Kundalini energy.

Kundalini's representation often involves intricate symbolism and imagery, contributing to its mystique. The coiled serpent is a recurring motif, symbolizing the latent potential within each individual. Additionally, Kundalini is depicted as a goddess, often named Shakti, symbolizing divine feminine energy. This symbolism reflects the union of Shiva, representing consciousness, with Shakti, representing energy, emphasizing the harmonious balance necessary for spiritual awakening.

Integrating Kundalini into various yoga practices has been a significant aspect of its historical evolution. Kundalini awakening can be approached holistically with yoga, a diverse practice that includes physical postures, breath control, and meditation. Kundalini Yoga focuses explicitly on techniques to stimulate and guide the ascending energy. Kundalini Yoga incorporates dynamic movements, breathwork (pranayama), and meditation, creating a comprehensive system to facilitate the awakening and harmonious flow of Kundalini energy.

While Kundalini is most commonly associated with Hinduism, echoes of similar concepts can be found in other Eastern traditions. In Buddhism, the concept of subtle energy channels, or nadis, parallels the idea of Kundalini's ascent through the Chakras. Additionally, Taoist alchemy in China explores internal energy cultivation, resembling the transformative processes associated with the Kundalini awakening. These cross-cultural connections highlight the universal spiritual power and transformation themes present in ancient wisdom traditions.

The journey of Kundalini awakening has challenges and risks. Many ancient texts emphasize the importance of a knowledgeable guide or guru to navigate the complexities of Kundalini experiences. Individuals may encounter physical, emotional, or psychological difficulties during the awakening process without proper guidance. The intensity of Kundalini experiences varies, and while some report profound spiritual insights and heightened awareness, others may face overwhelming sensations that can be disorienting.

In the 20th century, Kundalini experienced a resurgence of interest within the context of the New Age movement. Western spiritual seekers, drawn to Eastern philosophies, began exploring Kundalini as a pathway to higher consciousness and personal transformation. The teachings of spiritual leaders such as Swami Sivananda, Yogi Bhajan, and Gopi Krishna popularized Kundalini practices in the West. With its dynamic movements and emphasis on awakening dormant energy, Kundalini Yoga became a prominent form of yoga in Western countries.

While Kundalini is deeply rooted in spiritual and metaphysical traditions, some contemporary perspectives seek to understand its phenomena through a scientific lens. Neuroscientists and psychologists explore the physiological and psychological aspects of Kundalini's experiences, attempting to demystify the transformative processes associated with its awakening. Some researchers suggest that Kundalini's experiences may be linked to altered states of consciousness, neuroplasticity, and the release of certain neurotransmitters.

In summary, Kundalini's history and origins are intricately intertwined within the rich fabric of old Eastern traditions, where it first appeared as a profound idea that represents the innate spiritual force that lies dormant within each person. From its roots in Hinduism to its integration into Tantric practices, Kundalini has undergone a transformative journey, influencing various spiritual disciplines. The symbolism, imagery, and practices associated with Kundalini continue to captivate spiritual seekers in both traditional and modern contexts. As

Kundalini finds resonance in diverse cultural and spiritual landscapes, its exploration invites individuals to delve into the depths of their consciousness in pursuit of spiritual awakening and self-realization.

The nature of Kundalini energy

Spiritual traditions firmly hold kundalini energy, a mysterious power thought to lay dormant at the base of the spine. Studying Kundalini means exploring its esoteric core, its healing potential, and its significant influence on a person's spiritual development. This section delves into the nature of Kundalini's energy, looking at its traits, meanings, and the life-changing events that come with its awakening.

The nature of Kundalini is often symbolized by a coiled serpent residing at the Muladhara Chakra, located at the base of the spine in the human energy system. This symbolism is pervasive in Hindu and Tantric traditions, where the coiled serpent represents latent spiritual potential awaiting awakening. The serpent is both a powerful and primal symbol, embodying the cyclical nature of life, death, and rebirth. Additionally, Kundalini is often personified as a goddess, commonly known as Shakti, representing the divine feminine energy. The union of Shiva, symbolizing consciousness, with Shakti, indicating power, illustrates the harmonious balance required for spiritual awakening. The symbolism surrounding Kundalini emphasizes the transformative journey from dormancy to ascension, mirroring the cyclical patterns inherent in the natural world. Understanding the nature of Kundalini energy involves delving into the energetic anatomy of the human body, particularly the Chakra system. In H Hindu and yogic philosophy, Chakras are considered energy centers that align along the spine, each associated with specific qualities and aspects of human experience. At the base, the Muladhara Chakra is believed to be the seat of

Kundalini energy. As the dormant serpent awakens, it ascends through the Chakras, piercing each one and unleashing its transformative power. The Chakras serve as gateways for the flow of energy. Kundalini's awakening is thought to cleanse and activate these energy centers, leading to heightened consciousness and spiritual awakening.

The nature of Kundalini's energy is closely tied to its transformative potential. Awakening Kundalini is a profound and e-altering experience, leading to spiritual enlightenment and a deep connection with the divine. Intense physical, emotional, and spiritual experiences often mark the transformative journey. Practitioners describe experiencing heat, energy surges, vibrations, and heightened awareness of their inner selves. It is believed that once awakened, Kundalini energy elevates and purifies the individual's consciousness, enabling them to break free from the limitations of their ego and ascend to higher states of awareness. Kundalini is a unique and challenging transforming force, requiring a solid commitment to introspection and spiritual development. The nature of Kundalini is explored and harnessed through various yogic practices, with Kundalini Yoga being a specific discipline dedicated to awakening and channelling this potent energy. Kundalini Yoga incorporates dynamic movements, breathwork (pranayama), meditation, and chanting to stimulate and guide the ascending Kundalini energy. The techniques employed in Kundalini Yoga are designed to awaken the dormant serpent, encouraging its upward ascent through the Chakras. As practitioners engage in these practices, they aim to cultivate a heightened awareness and a direct experience of the transformative power of Kundalini energy.

While the transformative potential of Kundalini is profound, the nature of its awakening is not without challenges and risks. The intense energy released during Kundalini experiences can overwhelm individuals, leading to physical, emotional, and psychological difficulties. Some practitioners may face involuntary movements, passionate emotions, or altered states of consciousness that can be disorienting. Proper guidance from experienced teachers or gurus is emphasized in many spiritual traditions to navigate the challenges associated with Kundalini awakening. Without guidance, the transformative nature of Kundalini can become a double- edged sword, demanding a delicate balance between exploration and ensuring one's well-being.

The nature of Kundalini energy extends beyond individual practices and traditions, revealing interconnectedness and universal themes in various spiritual and mystical traditions. While Kundalini is prominently featured in Hinduism and Tantric traditions, echoes of similar concepts can be found in Buddhism, Taoism, and Western esoteric traditions. The universal themes of subtle energy, spiritual awakening, and the transformative journey are evident in the diverse ways different cultures and spiritual paths conceptualize and explore Kundalini. This interconnectedness suggests a shared recognition of the profound nature of human consciousness and its potential for expansion and evolution.

In the modern era, scientific explorations have sought to understand the nature of Kundalini's experiences through the lens of neuroscience and psychology. Researchers attempt to demystify the physiological and psychological aspects of Kundalini awakening, considering it a potential avenue for exploring altered states of consciousness. Some people suggest that neuroplasticity, alterations in brain activity, and the release of neurotransmitters could be connected to the profound sensations associated with Kundalini. The investigation shows a rising interest in bridging the gap between spiritual experiences and the empirical methods of scientific inquiry, even though the scientific understanding of Kundalini is still in its infancy.

In conclusion, the nature of Kundalini energy is a multifaceted and profound concept that transcends cultural, religious, and philosophical boundaries. Symbolized by the coiled serpent and represented as a transformative force, Kundalini embodies the potential for spiritual awakening and heightened consciousness. Whether explored through ancient Hindu and Tantric traditions, integrated into yogic practices like Kundalini Yoga, or considered from a scientific perspective, the essence of Kundalini invites individuals to embark on a transformative journey within. As the serpent awakens and ascends through the Chakras, the nature of Kundalini unfolds as a dynamic force connecting the individual with the universal aspects of consciousness and the boundless potential for spiritual evolution.

How Kundalini energy manifests in the body and mind

The manifestation of Kundalini's energy within the human body and mind is a captivating exploration into the depths of spiritual experience. Rooted in ancient traditions, Kundalini is believed to be a dormant force coiled at the base of the spine, waiting to ascend through the Chakras, unlocking profound transformations. This section delves into the intricate ways Kundalini's energy manifests, examining its impact on the physical, emotional, and mental dimensions of an individual's being. From the subtle currents within the energetic anatomy to the heightened states of consciousness, understanding how Kundalini manifests provides insight into the profound nature of spiritual awakening.

Kundalini energy follows specific energetic pathways within the body, particularly along the spine through the Chakras. As the energy ascends, it pierces through each Chakra, activating and purifying these energy centers.

The intricate dance of Kundalini through the energetic pathways corresponds to a transformative journey, with each Chakra representing different aspects of human experience. The Muladhara is associated with survival instincts, while the Sahasrara, the crown Chakra, is linked to higher consciousness. The manifestation of Kundalini, as it travels through these energy centers, brings about a profound integration of physical, emotional, and spiritual dimensions.

One of the most tangible manifestations of Kundalini energy is the array of physical sensations experienced by practitioners during its awakening. These sensations can vary widely and are often described as intense heat, vibrations, tingling, or a feeling of electric currents running through the body. As Kundalini rises, it stimulates the nervous system and activates dormant energy, creating a heightened awareness of the physical body. The energy may also lead to spontaneous movements or yoga-like postures, known as kriyas, as the body responds to the flow of Kundalini. These physical manifestations not only indicate the energy's awakening but also serve as a form of purification and balancing of the body's subtle energies.

Kundalini's manifestation extends beyond the physical realm, profoundly influencing the emotional landscape of the practitioner. As the energy ascends, it is believed to stir and release stored emotions and memories. This intense emotional release can lead to euphoria, bliss, or, conversely, the surfacing of long-buried traumas. The manifestation of Kundalini's energy is thus intertwined with emotional cleansing and healing, allowing practitioners to confront and process unresolved aspects of their psyche. While emotional release can be challenging, it is an essential aspect of the transformative journey, paving the way for a more profound connection with one's emotions and a more excellent inner balance.

At the core of Kundalini's manifestation is the expansion of consciousness, offering practitioners a direct experience of heightened awareness and spiritual insight. This heightened awareness goes beyond the ordinary perception of reality, allowing individuals to tap into deeper layers of insight, intuition, and spiritual understanding. The manifestation of Kundalini in the mind transcends the limitations of the ego, providing a direct connection to the universal aspects of consciousness. This expansion of consciousness is often described as a state of oneness, where the boundaries between the self and the external world dissolve, revealing a profound interconnectedness.

Kundalini's manifestation brings about a profound integration of dualities within the individual, reconciling opposites and fostering a sense of inner unity. The ascent of Kunda is often described as the union of Shiva and Shakti, symbolizing the merging of masculine and feminine energies within the practitioner. This integration extends to the reconciliation of light and shadow aspects of the self, leading to a more holistic understanding of one's being. The manifestation of Kundalini energy facilitates the harmonious balance of polarities, allowing individuals to embrace the full spectrum of their existence. This integration is not only transformative personally but also reflects the universal principle of balance and harmony inherent in Kundalini.

While the manifestation of Kundalini energy brings about transformative experiences, it is not devoid of challenges and shadow aspects. The intensified energies and the surfacing of deep-seated emotions can lead to discomfort, emotional turmoil, or even a sense of losing control. The shadow aspects, often called the "Kundalini syndrome," may manifest as physical or psychological difficulties, requiring careful navigation and support. The challenges associated with Kundalini's manifestation highlight the importance of proper guidance, emphasizing the role of experienced teachers or gurus to assist individuals in navigating the complexities of the awakening process.

The manifestation of Kundalini energy extends beyond the moments of heightened experiences during meditation or yoga practices. It gradually integrates into the practitioner's daily life, influencing perceptions, relationships, and decision-making. The expanded consciousness and heightened awareness attained through Kundalini's manifestation foster a more mindful and present way of living. Individuals may find themselves more attuned to the subtleties of their surroundings, cultivating a deep sense of gratitude and interconnectedness with the world. The integration of Kundalini into daily life is a testament to its transformative nature, influencing the internal landscape and the external expression of one's being.

In recent years, there has been a growing interest in understanding the manifestations of Kundalini energy from a scientific standpoint. Neuroscientists and psychologists explore the physiological and psychological changes associated with Kundalini experiences. Some researchers propose that the sensations and altered states of consciousness may be linked to changes in brain activity, the release of neurotransmitters, and neuroplasticity. While scientific perspectives are valuable in demystifying aspects of Kundalini manifestations, they also underscore the limitations of purely reductionist approaches in capturing the full spectrum of spiritual experiences.

In conclusion, the manifestations of Kundalini energy within the body and mind weave a complex tapestry of experiences, transcending the boundaries between human existence and physical, emotional, and spiritual dimensions. From the subtle currents along the energetic pathways to the profound expansion of consciousness, Kundalini's impact is transformative and multifaceted.

The physical sensations, emotional release, and integration of dualities contribute to the profound journey of self-discovery and spiritual awakening. One can better understand oneself and the interconnectedness of all existence by embracing the shadow parts and navigating the challenges presented by Kundalini manifestations. This exploration invites people to go on a transformative journey that goes beyond the limits of conventional understanding by fusing the ancient wisdom of Kundalini with modern scientific study.

CHAPTER II

The Chakra System

An in-depth look at the seven chakras

An in-depth exploration of the chakras offers a profound understanding of the subtle energy centres integral to various spiritual and healing traditions. Chakras, named after the Sanskrit word for "wheel" or "disk," are thought to be whirling energy vortices inside the human energy field. Each chakra is associated with specific qualities, attributes, and aspects of the human experience, contributing to an individual's overall balance and well-being. The concept of chakras originates from ancient Indian spiritual practices, particularly within the tradition of yoga and the system of Ayurveda. In this section, we delve into the characteristics, functions, and significance of each of the seven chakras, unravelling the intricate web of energy that connects human existence's physical, mental, and spiritual dimensions.

The first chakra, known as the Root Chakra or Mujadara, is at the spine's base and associated with red. As the foundation of the chakra system, Mujadara represents stability, security, and the primal connection to the physical world. It governs basic survival needs like food, shelter, and safety. When the Root Chakra is balanced, individuals feel grounded, secure, and connected to the Earth. This chakra imbalance may manifest as fear, insecurity, or instability.

Moving up the chakra system, the second chakra is the Sacral Chakra, or Vibhishana, located in the lower abdomen and associated with orange. This chakra gives creativity, sensuality, emotion, and well-being. A balanced Sacral Chakra fosters a sense of pleasure, joy, and emotional resilience. Unbalance can result in a lack of passion, emotional instability, or creative difficulties. The Sacral Chakra can be energized and harmonized through activities such as dance, artistic expression, and working with orange crystals like carnelian.

The centre of one's strength, determination, and self-worth is this chakra. This chakra is the centre of personal power, will, and self-esteem. It governs the digestive system and is linked to the element of fire. A balanced Solar Plexus Chak empowers individuals to assert themselves, set healthy boundaries, and confidently pursue their goals. Imbalances in this chakra may manifest as feelings of powerlessness, low self-esteem, or digestive issues. Practices such as mindful breathing, core strengthening exercises, and yellow crystals like Citrine can help balance and activate the Solar Plexus Chakra. The

Heart Chakra governs love, compassion, and emotional balance as the bridge between the low and upper chakras. It is linked to the air element, symbolizing the breath of life and interconnectedness. A balanced Heart Chakra allows for open-hearted connections, empathy, and harmony. Imbalances may manifest as issues with trust, emotional coldness, or difficulty forming healthy relationships. Practice such as heart-opening y ga poses, a meditation on compassion, and working with heart-cantered crystals like rose quartz can support the balance of the Heart Chakra.

It is located in the throat area and is connected to blue. This chakra governs communication, self-expression, and the ability to speak one's truth. It's linked to the element of sound, emphasizing the power of said words. A balanced Throat Chakra enables clear and authentic communication, while imbalances may result in difficulty expressing oneself, throat-related ailments, or a fear of speaking up. Practices like chanting, singing, and using throat-chakra crystals like aquamarine or blue lace agate can help activate and align the Throat Chakra.

This chakra governs intuition, perception, and inner wisdom. Often referred to as the "seat of the soul," the Third Eye Chakra is linked to the element of light and the pineal gland. A balanced Third Eye Chakra enhances intuitive abilities, insight, and clarity of thought. Imbalances may manifest as confusion, lack of focus, or a disconnection from inner guidance. Practices like meditation, visualization, and working with go crystals like lapis lazuli or amethyst can help activate and attune the Third Eye Chakra.

This chakra represents so ritual connection, divine consciousness, and the integration of all aspects of the self. The Crown Chak is often considered the gateway to higher awareness and enlightenment. A balanced Crown Chakra allows individuals to experience a sense of unity with the universe and a profound connection to the divine. Imbalances may result in feelings of disconnection, spiritual apathy, or an attachment to worldly pursuits. Practices such as meditation, prayer, and working with crown-chakra crystals like clear quartz or amethyst can support the activation and alignment of the Crown Chakra.

The interconnected ess of the seven chakras forms a dynamic system that reflects the holistic nature of human experience. The general equilibrium of the system as a whole and the health of each particular chakra affect how energy moves through the energy centres. Many techniques, including energy healing, crystal treatment, yoga, and meditation, aim to keep the chakras working in a harmonic manner. Through knowledge of the characteristics of each chakra, people can set out on a path of self-discovery, healing, and spiritual enlightenment.

Moreover, the chakra system serves as a bridge between the physical and energetic dimensions of human existence. It provides a framework for understanding the intricate interplay between the body, mind, and spirit. Balancing and aligning the chakras promotes overall well-being, enhances vitality, and contributes to a more harmonious and fulfilling life. While chakras originate from ancient spiritual traditions, their relevance endures as individuals seek holistic approaches to health and self-realization in the modern world.

In conclusion, exploring the seven chakras unveils a fascinating tapestry of energy centres that intricately shape the human experience. From the foundational stability of the Root Chakra to the expansive awareness of the Crown Chakra, each chakra contributes to the holistic well-being of an individual. The journey through the chakras involves a continuous process of self-awareness, healing, and spiritual evolution. People can go on a journey of transformation that balances their energetic, emotional, and spiritual aspects and fosters a deeper connection to the great mysteries of creation by learning about each chakra's properties, functions, and significance.

Understanding the role of each chakra in Kundalini awakening

Understanding the role of each chakra in Kundalini's awakening unveils a profound journey of spiritual evolution and self-realization. Kundalini, a Sanskrit term for "coiled serpent," refers to the dormant spiritual energy believed to reside at the base of the spine. The awakening of Kundalini is often described as the ascent of this energy through the central energy channel, or Sushumna, which is intricately connected to the seven chakras. Every chakra acts as a centre for particular facets of awareness, and the enlightenment, union with the divine, and elevated awareness that come with Kundalini awakening are described. This section traces the path of this powerful spiritual energy from the base to the top of the energetic spine, examining the distinct roles that each chakra performs in the Kundalini awakening process.

The journey begins with the Root Chakra, Mujadara, situated at the base of the spine. Symbolized by a vibrant red colour, Mujadara is associated with the primal forces of survival, grounding, and connection to the physical world. In Kundalini's awakening, the dormant serpent energy is said to reside in this foundational chakra, coiled and waiting for the transformative journey ahead. The opening and activation of the Root Chakra lay the groundwork for Kundalini to begin its ascension, establishing a sense of stability, security, and connection to the earthly realm. Practices such as grounding meditations, visualization, and mindful awareness of the b dy contribute to the initial awakening of Kundalini at the Root Chakra.

Moving to the second chakra, Vibhishana, or the Sacral Chakra, Kundalini's journey involves exploring creativity, sensuality, and emotional fluidity. Vibhishana is often represented by the colour orange and is associated with the element of water. As Kundalini's energy rises, exploring emotions, relationships, and creative expression becomes a focal point. The awakening at the Sacral Chakra invites individuals to embrace their sensual and innovative nature, fostering a deeper connection to the ebb and flow of life's experiences. Practices such as artistic expression, dan e, and emotional release contribute to the activation of Kundalini at the Sacral Chakra.

The Solar Plexus Chakra, Manipura, located in the upper abdomen and radiates bright yellow energy, is activated next in the climb. This chakra controls one's will, power, and sense of identity. Kundalini's awakening at Manipura involves transforming one's sense of identity and empowerment. As the serpent energy rises to the Solar Plexus, individuals may experience a heightened sense of personal will, confidence, and the ability to manifest their intentions. Practices such as breathwork, empowerment exercises, and mindful self-reflection contribute to the activation of Kundalini at the Solar Plexus Chakra.

As Kundalini energy unfolds at the Heart Chakra, individuals enter a profound love, compassion, and interconnectedness realm. The weakened ng at Anahata invites individuals to transcend personal boundaries and embrace a universal love that extends beyond the self. Compassion towards oneself and others becomes critical to the Kundalini journey at the Heart Chakra. Practices such as heart-centred meditation, acts of kindness, and heart-opening yoga postures contribute to the activation of Kundalini in this expansive and transformative centre.

Continuing its ascent, Kundalini reaches the Throat Chakra, Vasudha, represented by a bright blue colour. The awakening at the Throat Chakra involves the expression of authentic truth, clear communication, and aligning one's words with the divine pose. As Kundalini energizes Vasudha, individuals may experience a deepening of their ability to speak their truth and communicate with clarity. The Third at Chakra becomes a portal for expressing divine wisdom and manifesting higher truths. Practices such as chanting, singing, and conscious communication contribute to the activation of Kundalini at the Throat Chakra.

The journey unfolds further by activating the Third Eye Chakra, Ajna, which is located between the eyebrows and is often associated with indigo. Kundalini's awakening at Ajn involves the expansion of intuitive abilities, inner vision, and heightened states of consciousness. As the serpent energy ends in the Third year, individuals may experience increased clarity, insight, and a connection to higher realms of awareness. The Third Eye Chakra becomes a gateway to spiritual vision and inner knowing. Practices such as meditation, visualization, and third-party awakening techniques contribute to the activation of Kundalini at Ajna.

The culmination of the Kundalini journey is at the Crown Chakra, sahasrara, situated at the top of the head and symbolized by a violet or white color. The opening of the Crown Chakra represents the union of individual consciousness with universal consciousness, the divine, and the infinite. Kunalini's awakening at Sahasra leads to spiritual bliss, transcendence, and a profound sense of unity with all existence. The Crown Chakra becomes the gateway to higher awareness and realizing one's divine nature. Practices such as meditation, prayer, and surrender to the divine contribute to the activation of Kundalini at the Crown Chakra.

Throughout this journey, the role of each chakra in Kundalini awakening is distinct and significant. The chakras serve as energetic gateways through which the serpent energy ascends, bringing about a profound transformation of consciousness and spiritual awakening. The balanced activation of all se en chakras allows for the harmonious flow of Kundalini energy, fostering a state of equilibrium and unity within the individual.

It is essential to approach Kundalini's awakening with reverence, mindfulness, and a deep understanding of its transformative power. While the journey can be enriching, it may also bring challenges and the need for a grounded and supportive spiritual practice. Seeking guidance from experienced teachers, engaging in practices that support energetic balance, and honouring the individual pace of the Kundalini journey are crucial aspects of navigating this profound awakening.

In conclusion, understanding each chakra's role in K kundalini's awakening provides a roadmap for individuals on spiritual evolution. The journey from the Root Chakra to the Crown Chakra involves the activation and harmonization of each energy centre, paving the way for the ascent of Kundalini energy. A deeper connection to oneself, others, and the divine may be found when people set out on this life-changing path, and they may also undergo the profound changes that come with the waking of the coiled serpent inside.

Techniques for balancing and aligning the chakras

Balancing and aligning the chakras is a holistic practice that seeks to harmonize energy flow within the body, mind, and spirit. The concept of chakras, originating from ancient Indian traditions, posits that these spinning energy centers influence various aspects of our well- being. When the chakras are balanced and aligned, they contribute to physical health, emotional stability, and spiritual awakening. This section explores various techniques that individuals can incorporate into their daily lives to foster the balance and alignment of the chakras. One fundamental technique for chakra balancing is meditation. Meditation provides a quiet space for self- reflection and inner exploration. Individuals can identify areas of imbalance by focusing on Ach chakra and inviting healing energy to those specific energy enter. Visualization during meditation, such as imagining a radiant light circulating through each chakra, is a powerful method for promoting alignment. Consistent meditation practice not only calms the mind but also supports the overall vitality and balance of the chakras.

Breathwork is another potent technique involving intentional breath control influencing energy flow. Pranayama, the yogic practice of breath control, offers various techniques that target specific chakras. For example, deep diaphragmatic breathing can help balance the Root Chakra, while al alternate nostril breathing may harmonize the energies of the Third Eye and Crown Chakras. Conscious breathing oxygenates the body and clears energetic blockages, facilitating the free flow of prana, or life force energy, through the chalk.

Yoga, integrating physical postures, breath control, and meditation, is a comprehensive practice for chakra balancing. Each yoga pose corresponds to specific chakras, helping to release tension and stimulate energy flow. Heart-opening poses like Cam l or Cobra ben fit the Heart Chakra while grounding poses like Mountain or Tree support the Root Chakra. The holistic nature of yoga makes it an effective tool for promoting overall chakra alignment and balance.

Another method that harmonizes with the chakras' vibrational frequencies is sound therapy. Bija mantras, or distinct sounds, are linked to each chakra. The chakras can be brought into harmony by chanting these mantras while in meditation or by employing singing bowls tuned to the appropriate frequencies. Sound has a profound vibratory impact that opens up the energy centers and encourages balance and harmony. Sound therapy takes the chakras on a sonic journey, which invites them to realign and rebalance their ideal frequencies.

Because of their energy qualities, crystals and gemstones have long been used, and they are essential for chakra balancing. Particular stones that resonate with the distinct energy of each chakra are linked to it. For instance, citrine corresponds with the solar plexus chakra, but amethyst is frequently used for crown chakra.

Another method for balancing the chakras is aromatherapy, which uses the power of essential oils. Certain fragrances can energize or calm the energy centers; each aroma corresponds to a particular chakra. For example, lavender is linked to the Crown Chakra, which fosters peace and spirituality. Chakra alignment can be achieved through a multisensory approach by using essential oils topically, diffusing them, or incorporating them into meditation activities.

Massage and bodywork contribute to chakra Bala by releasing physical and energetic tension stored in the body. Techniques like acupressure, reflexology, or Reiki can target specific chakras, promoting relaxation and facilitating energy flow. Massage addresses physical tension and works subtly to harmonize the energetic imbalances within the chakra system.

Color therapy, or chromotherapy, involves exposure to specific colors to influence the energy centers. Each chakra is associated with a particular color, and incorporating these has into one's environment or clothing can have a balancing effect. Visualization of vibrant colors during meditation or using colored filters in lighting are additional ways to engage in color therapy for chakra alignment.

Movement practices, such as dance or tai hi, offer dynamic approaches to chakra balancing. These practices' rhythmic and flowing movements stimulate the energy centers, encouraging the release of stagnant energy and promoting a sense of vitality. In dance, expressive movement allows people to connect with their emotions and let go of energetic obstructions that could interfere with the chakras.

The connection to nature offers a straightforward yet effective method for balancing the chakras. Walking in the woods, relaxing by the sea, or just taking in the beauty of the natural world may all be peaceful, reviving experiences for the chakras. People can be gently reminded to tune into the natural cycles of energy flow within their bodies by nature's innate balance and harmony.

Mindfulness practices, such as conscious eating or mindful walking, contribute to Balancing Chakra by tearing present-moment awareness. By bringing attention to daily activities, individuals can become attuned to the energetic qualities associated with each chakra. Mindful practices help prevent the accumulation of stress and tension, supporting the overall health and equilibrium of the chakra system.

Chakra rebalancing and alignment are achieved by channelling healing energy, as in energy healing therapies like Qi Gong and Reiki. Practitioners employ practical procedures that guide energy flow to correct imbalances within the energy centers. Energy healing sessions benefit people looking for a more focused and direct method of balancing their chakras.

Journaling serves as a reflective practice for chakra awareness and alignment. Keeping a chakra journal allows individuals to track their thoughts, emotions, and experiences related to each energy cycle. Individuals can implement targeted practices to address specific chakra imbalances by identifying patterns and areas of concern. Journaling also provides a valuable tool for self-discovery and self-healing.

Holistic therapies, such as Ayurveda or Traditional Chinese Medicine (TCM), offer comprehensive approaches to balancing chakra by addressing physical, emotional, energetic, and well-being. These systems recognize the connectedness of various elements in the body and provide personalized recommendations, including dietary changes, herbal remedies, and lifestyle adjustments to support chakra harmony.

In conclusion, the techniques for balancing and aligning the chakras are diverse and adaptable, catering to individual preferences and needs. The holistic nature of these practices recognizes the intricate interplay between the physical, emotional, and spiritual dimensions of well-being. Whether through meditation, breathwork, yoga, or other modalities, individuals can explore and integrate these techniques to foster a harmonious flow of energy within the chakra system. People who set out on this path of self-awareness and energetic equilibrium expose themselves to the life-changing power of chakra alignment, feeling more alive, resilient emotionally, and experiencing spiritual awakening.

CHAPTER III

Signs and Symptoms of Kundalini Awakening

Recognizing the early signs of Kundalini activation

Recognizing the early signs of Kundalini activation marks the beginning of a profound spiritual journey. Many ancient traditions, especially those related to yoga and meditation, have highly valued and utilized this method. Kundalini, frequently seen at the base of the spine as a coiling serpent, symbolizes spiritual energy that is asleep and needs to awaken. People may feel a variety of subtle yet transformational indicators when this powerful force starts to stir, providing a look into the incredible journey ahead. Understanding and acknowledging these early signs is essential for those treading the path of Kundalini awakening, as it brings awareness to the subtle shifts occurring within the physical, mental, and energetic dimensions.

One of the initial signs of Kundalini activation is heightened physical and emotional sensitivity. Individuals may find themselves more attuned to their surroundings, experiencing a heightened awareness of sensory stimuli. Sounds may sound louder, emotions more tangible, and colors more vivid. The expansion of consciousness and the awakening of the subtle energy body that accompanies Kundalini activation is reflected in this enhanced sensitivity. People may experience an improved sense of the interconnection of everything as the energy rises, promoting a sense of oneness with the surroundings.

A notable physical manifestation of early Kundalini activation is the sensation of energy movements within the body. This may manifest as tingling, warmth, or gentle electric currents moving along the spine or through various energy centers. These sensations indicate the Kundalini energy beginning to ascend through the central channel or Sushumna. Individuals may feel pulsating energy, like a rhythmic heartbeat, as the dormant serpent gradually stirs to life. These physical sensations serve as tangible reminders of the energetic shifts occurring within, signaling the initiation of a transformative process.

Heightened and altered states of awareness are common precursors to Kundalini activation. Individuals may experience vivid dreams, lucid states, or a deepening of meditation experiences. The thinning of the veil between the conscious and subconscious mind results from the Kundalini energy influencing the higher centers of consciousness. Such experiences offer glimpses into expanded states of awareness, providing a taste of the spiritual insights and revelations that may unfold as the Kundalini journey progresses.

As Kundalini activation progresses, individuals may encounter spontaneous movements or kriyas. These involuntary bodily movements, such as spontaneous yoga postures, shaking, or trembling, are natural expressions of the rising Kundalini energy. The body intuitively adjusts to accommodate the increased energy flow, releasing accumulated tension or blockages. While these movements may initially be surprising, they are an integral part of the transformative process, aiding in the purification and realignment of the energy centers. Psychological and emotional shifts are also prominent early signs of Kundalini activation. Individuals may undergo periods of introspection, self-inquiry, or a deepening of their spiritual quest. The awakening Kundalini energy brings buried emotions and unresolved issues to the surface for healing and integration. Emotional releases, such as sudden bouts of laughter or tears, may occur as the Kundalini works to purify the emotional body. This phase of self-discovery and emotional clearing is an essential aspect of Kundalini's awakening, facilitating the evolution of consciousness and a deepening connection to one's innermost self.

Another significant indicator is the opening of the heart center. As the Kundalini energy rises, individuals may experience a profound shift in their capacity for love, compassion, and empathy. The heart center, or Anahata Chakra, radiates an enhanced sense of universal love, fostering a deep connection to all living beings. This heart chakra expansion is a pivotal aspect of Kundalini activation, leading to a more heart-centered and inclusive way of relating to the world.

Increased intuition and heightened psychic abilities often accompany early Kundalini activation. Individuals may find themselves more attuned to subtle energies, experiencing heightened intuition, clairvoyance, or telepathic abilities. This expansion of psychic faculties is a natural outcome of the Kundalini energy influencing the Third Eye Chakra, located between the eyebrows. As the third eye opens, individuals gain access to higher levels of perception and insight, guiding them on their spiritual path.

While these signs of Kundalini activation indicate a transformative process, it is crucial to approach the journey with mindfulness and self-awareness. The intensity and nature of Kundalini experiences vary among individuals, and what may be a harmonious awakening for one person could pose challenges for another. To make the trip via support and understanding, it is recommended that persons undergoing Kundalini activation seek direction from knowledgeable teachers, mentors, or spiritual communities.

Though subtle, the early signs of Kundalini activation lay the foundation for a profound and transformative journey. Recognizing and embracing these signs allows individuals to consciously participate in awakening, fostering a harmonious alignment of the physical, mental, and energetic dimensions. As the Kundalini energy continues its ascent, individuals may undergo further purification, revelation, and spiritual growth, ultimately leading to heightened awareness, inner illumination, and a deepened connection to the divine within and beyond.

Common physical, emotional, and spiritual symptoms

A profound spiritual journey with ancient roots, kundalini awakening, entails reawakening latent spiritual energy thought to be located at the base of the spine. People frequently experience a range of physical, emotional, and spiritual symptoms that indicate the transformational character of this awakening process as this powerful force ascends through the primary energy channel.

Physically, Kundalini awakening is frequently accompanied by distinctive sensations that indicate the activation and movement of energy within the body. Many individuals report feeling tingling, warmth, or gentle electric currents along the spine or through the chakras, the energy centers aligned along the spinal column. These sensations are tangible expressions of the Kundalini energy rising from its dormant state. As the energy moves, individuals may also experience spontaneous physical movements or kriyas, including yoga postures, shaking, or trembling. These movements are considered natural responses to the heightened energy flow and are crucial in releasing tension and energetic blockages within the body.

Furthermore, a Kundalini awakening can alter sensory perception, which can show up as an increased level of environmental awareness. Sounds may seem more resonant, colors more vivid, and subtle energy flows may become more apparent. The expanded awareness linked to Kundalini activation is reflected in this sensory increase. The physical body adjusts to the increased energetic activity caused by the rising Kundalini through a purifying and adjustment process.

Emotionally, Kundalini's awakening often stirs the depths of the emotional body, bringing forth a range of intense feelings and experiences. Emotional releases, such as sudden laughter, tears, or mood swings, are expected as the Kundalini energy works to purify and cleanse the dynamic landscape. Past traumas and unresolved emotions may surface, providing healing and integration opportunities. It is not unusual for individuals to undergo periods of profound bliss, joy, or ecstasy, reflecting a deepening connection to the divine and the transformative nature of the emotional shifts occurring during Kundalini's awakening.

However, the emotional aspect of Kundalini's awakening may also present challenges. Heightened emotional states, including fear, anxiety, or a sense of emotional overwhelm, can arise as the Kundalini energy works through layers of emotional blockages. It is crucial for individuals undergoing this process to approach their emotions with compassion and self-awareness, recognizing them as part of the purification and healing journey. Seeking therapeutic support or engaging in practices that promote emotional well-being can be beneficial during these phases.

Spiritually, Kundalini's awakening unfolds as a profound spiritual journey, leading to expanded states of consciousness and a deepened connection to the divine. One of the significant spiritual symptoms is the opening of the Third Eye Chakra, located between the eyebrows. This awakening is often accompanied by heightened intuition, clairvoyance, and a deeper perception of subtle energies. As the Kundalini energy ascends to the Crown Chakra at the top of the head, individuals may experience unity consciousness, a profound sense of oneness with the universe, and a deep inner peace.

The spiritual dimension of Kundalini's awakening also involves a process of self-discovery and a quest for deeper meaning. Individuals may undergo periods of introspection, self-inquiry, and a deepening connection to their spiritual essence. The expanded awareness and connection to higher states of consciousness contribute to a sense of purpose and a profound shift in one's understanding of the nature of reality.

Despite the transformative nature of Kundalini's awakening, individuals may encounter challenges on the spiritual plane. The heightened sensitivity to energies and expanded states of consciousness can lead to sensory overload or spiritual overwhelm. Maintaining a grounded and supportive environment, along with practices that promote spiritual integration, is essential for navigating the spiritual aspects of Kundalini awakening.

Sleep disruptions are another common aspect of Kundalini awakening, impacting the individual's dream state and overall sleep patterns. Vivid dreams, lucid states, or altered states of consciousness during sleep are common occurrences. These experiences often reflect deep inner processing and spiritual insights due to Kundalini's energy's influence on the subconscious mind. Creating a conducive sleep environment, practicing relaxation techniques, and maintaining a consistent sleep routine can support individuals in managing sleep disturbances during the awakening process.

Physical sensations of heat or energy surges, particularly along the spine or in the palms of the hands, are prevalent symptoms of Kundalini awakening. The increased energy flow may create a sense of warmth, tingling, or vibrations in specific body areas. These sensations indicate the activation of energy centers and the alignment of the Kundalini energy. Individuals may also experience an expansion of the energy field, a palpable radiance or aura surrounding the body, signifying the heightened vibrational frequency associated with Kundalini activation.

Gastrointestinal disturbances, such as changes in appetite, digestion, or elimination patterns, can occur during Kundalini awakening. The increased energy flow affects the functioning of the digestive organs, and individuals may notice shifts in their dietary preferences or a heightened awareness of the energetic qualities of food. Maintaining a balanced and nourishing diet and staying hydrated supports the physical body in adapting to the changes brought about by Kundalini activation.

In conclusion, the symptoms of Kundalini's awakening encompass a diverse range of physical, emotional, and spiritual experiences, all integral to this profound journey's transformative nature. As individuals traverse the various dimensions of Kundalini activation, they are invited to cultivate self-awareness, resilience, and a deepened connection to their innermost being. Seeking guidance from experienced mentors, teachers, or spiritual communities can provide valuable support, aiding individuals in navigating the challenges and embracing the profound possibilities accompanying Kundalini's awakening.

Navigating the challenges of Kundalini awakening

Navigating the challenges of Kundalini awakening is an integral aspect of the profound spiritual journey that unfolds when the dormant spiritual energy at the base of the spine is activated. While Kundalini's awakening holds the promise of expanded consciousness, spiritual insight, and transformative growth, it is not without its difficulties. Individuals undergoing this awakening may encounter various physical and psychological challenges as the potent Kundalini energy works through the multiple layers of the being.

One of the primary challenges during Kundalini awakening is the intensity of the energetic experiences. The heightened energy flow along the spine and through the chakras can be overwhelming, leading to sensations of heat, tingling, or even electric currents. These intense, energetic shifts may cause discomfort or anxiety, especially for those unprepared or unfamiliar with the sensations associated with Kundalini activation. Individuals need to cultivate self-awareness and a sense of grounding to navigate these intense, energetic experiences effectively.

Physical discomfort is a common challenge during Kundalini awakening. Individuals may experience symptoms such as headaches, muscle spasms, or fatigue as the energy moves through the body and releases stored tension. The physical body undergoes a purification process, adjusting to the increased vibrational frequency brought about by Kundalini activation. Individuals must engage in practices that support physical well-being, including regular exercise, proper nutrition, and adequate rest. Seeking guidance from healthcare professionals can also provide reassurance and address any concerns related to physical symptoms.

Psychological challenges often arise as Kundalini energy works through the emotional and mental realms. Intense emotional releases, including bouts of laughter, tears, or mood swings, can be disconcerting for individuals navigating the dynamic landscape of the awakening process. Past traumas and unresolved emotions may surface, requiring careful and compassionate attention. Psychological support through therapy, counseling, or engaging in practices that promote emotional well-being can be crucial for managing the psychological challenges associated with Kundalini awakening.

Another significant challenge is the potential for spiritual overwhelm. Heightened states of consciousness, expanded awareness and encounters with spiritual dimensions can be profound but may also be disorienting for individuals unaccustomed to such experiences. Spiritual overload can lead to confusion, disconnection from everyday reality, or difficulty integrating spiritual insights into daily life. People can overcome spiritual overwhelm by adopting a balanced approach to spiritual development, including grounding techniques and consulting with knowledgeable spiritual mentors.

One of the most prevalent challenges during Kundalini awakening is sleep disturbance. The Kundalini energy affects the subconscious mind, leading to vivid dreams, altered states of consciousness, or irregular sleep patterns. Although these encounters can provide insightful information and spiritual direction, they may also hurt the general sleep quality. People can manage sleep problems during awakening by practicing relaxation techniques, making a favorable sleep environment, and establishing a regular and peaceful nighttime.

Social and interpersonal challenges may arise as individuals undergo profound changes during Kundalini's awakening. Shifts in values, perspectives, and priorities can impact relationships with family, friends, or the larger community. Individuals may struggle to articulate their spiritual experiences or feel isolated if those around them need help understanding or sharing similar perspectives. Building a supportive network of like-minded individuals, participating in spiritual communities, or seeking guidance from mentors can help individuals navigate the social and interpersonal aspects of Kundalini Awakening.

Integrating—harmonizing the experiences and insights gained during Kundalini's awakening into daily life is a crucial challenge. Integrating profound spiritual experiences into one's identity, work, and relationships requires a conscious and deliberate effort. Individuals may struggle to balance the expanded states of consciousness and the practical demands of everyday life. Developing a holistic approach to integration, incorporating spiritual practices into daily routines, and maintaining a sense of self-care are essential to navigating the integration challenges associated with Kundalini awakening.

Another significant challenge is the potential for overemphasis on the experiences themselves. The extraordinary nature of Kundalini's awakening experiences may make individuals overly focused on pursuing transcendent states, spiritual phenomena, or mystical encounters. This overemphasis on the special may result in a neglect of the grounded and practical aspects of daily life. Individuals need to maintain a balanced approach, recognizing that spiritual growth involves transcendent experiences and the integration of those experiences into the fabric of everyday existence.

Fear and resistance can emerge as formidable challenges during Kundalini's awakening. The unknown nature of the process, coupled with intense energetic experiences, may trigger fear or resistance within individuals. Fear of losing control, fear of the novel, or fear of facing unresolved aspects of the self can create barriers to the smooth progression of Kundalini awakening. Individuals need to cultivate a mindset of openness, surrender, and trust in the inherent wisdom of the awakening process. Mindfulness, meditation, and self-inquiry can help individuals navigate and transcend fear and resistance. In

conclusion, navigating the challenges of Kundalini awakening is a dynamic and individualized journey that requires mindful awareness, resilience, and a holistic approach to well-being. Recognizing that challenges are inherent to the transformative nature of the awakening process allows individuals to approach difficulties with a sense of curiosity and openness. Seeking guidance from experienced mentors, engaging in supportive communities, and incorporating holistic practices can provide valuable resources for those undergoing Kundalini awakening. As individuals courageously navigate the challenges, they unlock the profound potential for spiritual growth, self-discovery, and a deepened connection to the expansive realms of consciousness.

CHAPTER IV

Preparation for Kundalini Awakening

Mind-body practices for preparing the system

The activation of dormant spiritual energy at the base of the spine, known as Kundalini awakening, is a deep and transforming process made possible via mind-body activities. These methods, which originated in ancient wisdom and other cultural traditions, provide a comprehensive way to develop a balanced alignment of the person's mental, bodily, and energetic aspects. These practices generate a condition of mind and body balance and receptivity that facilitates the smooth and aware unfolding of the Kundalini awakening process.

Meditation is at the forefront when it comes to mind-body techniques that prime the body for Kundalini awakening. Meditation is a valuable tool for improving self-awareness, calming the mind, and promoting inner serenity via mindfulness and focused attention. Frequent meditation establishes a solid mental foundation that enables people to observe their feelings, ideas, and experiences objectively. As Kundalini energy rises, people benefit significantly from this mental clarity because it makes them more capable of handling subtle energetic shifts and elevated consciousness.

Yoga is a comprehensive mind-body discipline that originated in India and consists of physical postures called asanas, breath control techniques called pranayama, and meditation. Specific yoga asanas are designed to activate and balance the energy centers or chakras, preparing the energetic pathways for the upward movement of Kundalini energy. Pranayama, or breathwork, is integral in regulating the breath, increasing pranic (life force) power, and promoting a state of calm receptivity—essential elements for Kundalini's safe and effective awakening.

Tai Chi and Qigong are ancient Chinese mind-body practices emphasizing the cultivation and circulation of vital energy, known as Qi or Chi. These gentle, flowing movements, combined with focused breathwork and meditative awareness, enhance the body's balance and flow of energy. By fostering a sense of relaxation and fluidity, Tai Chi and Qigong contribute to the overall energetic preparation of the system for Kundalini awakening. The slow, deliberate movements also ground the practitioner, promoting a deep connection to the earth—an essential aspect as the Kundalini energy rises.

Regardless of particular yoga postures, breathwork is extremely important for setting up the body for Kundalini activation. Numerous breathwork methods improve oxygenation and life force energy flow, including deep diaphragmatic breathing, alternate nostril breathing (Nadi Shodhana), and breath retention (Kumbhaka). By regulating the autonomic nervous system, conscious control of breathing can induce a sense of calm and relaxation. Intentional and rhythmic breathing practices provide an ideal basis for the awakening process because Kundalini's energy is particularly sensitive to the quality of breath.

Mindfulness Practices, including mindful awareness and present-moment attention, are essential to preparing the mind for Kundalini awakening. Cultivating an attentive and non-judgmental awareness of thoughts, emotions, and sensations allows individuals to develop resilience and stability in the face of intense experiences. Mindfulness practices also foster a deepened connection to the present moment, anchoring individuals in the now and reducing the influence of past and future concerns—

an invaluable resource during the transformative journey of Kundalini's awakening.

Visualization Techniques harness the power of the mind to direct energy and intention, contributing to the preparatory phase for Kundalini awakening. Visualization practices involve creating mental images or scenarios that align with the desired outcomes of the awakening process. For example, visualizing the smooth and upward flow of a coiled serpent (representing Kundalini energy) through the chakras can enhance the receptivity of the energy centers. Visualization bridges the mental and energetic realms, establishing a coherent and intentional framework for the unfolding Kundalini journey.

Sound Healing through practices like chanting, mantra repetition, or exposure to specific frequencies contributes to the vibrational preparation of the system for Kundalini awakening. Sound profoundly impacts the subtle energy body, resonating with and harmonizing the chakras. Chanting specific mantras, such as the universal "Om," activates the throat and crown chakras, aligning the practitioner with higher states of consciousness. Sound healing induces a resonance within the energetic field, attuning the individual to frequencies that support the safe and gradual ascent of Kundalini energy.

Incorporating these mind-body practices into a holistic preparatory routine creates a synergistic effect, fostering a balanced and receptive state within the individual. Integrating meditation, yoga, breathwork, Tai Chi, Qigong, mindfulness practices, visualization, and sound healing collectively creates a foundation that supports the gradual awakening and ascent of Kundalini energy.

It is crucial to approach these practices with an attitude of openness, patience, and respect for each individual's unique journey. Kundalini awakening is a highly individualized process, and the preparatory phase sets the stage for a conscious and harmonious unfolding.

Seeking guidance from experienced teachers, mentors, or spiritual communities can provide valuable support and insights during this preparatory phase, ensuring that individuals embark on their Kundalini journey with mindfulness, readiness, and a profound connection to the transformative power within.

Cultivating mindfulness and self-awareness

To navigate the dramatic and transformative experience of awakening dormant spiritual energy at the base of the spine, one must cultivate self-awareness and mindfulness during Kundalini's awakening. With its origins in ancient contemplative traditions, mindfulness is constantly being objectively aware of one's thoughts, feelings, sensations, and surroundings. This deliberate and non-reactive presence is a guiding light throughout the waking process, promoting a more profound comprehension of oneself and the subtleties of the energetic shifts connected to Kundalini activation.

Mindfulness Practices: Central to cultivating mindfulness during Kundalini awakening are various mindfulness practices that bring attention to the present moment. Mindful breathing, where individuals focus on the inhalation and exhalation of the breath, is a foundational practice. The breath becomes an anchor, grounding individuals in the immediacy of each moment. Mindful walking, eating, and daily activities encourage a heightened awareness of the body's movements and sensations, promoting a conscious presence.

Observation of Thoughts and Emotions: An essential aspect of mindfulness during Kundalini's awakening involves observing thoughts and emotions with a detached yet compassionate awareness. The intense energetic shifts may give rise to various emotions and thoughts, from blissful states to challenging emotional releases. Mindful observation allows individuals to witness these mental and emotional phenomena without becoming entangled. This non-attachment creates a spacious mental environment accommodating the ebb and flow of inner experiences.

Body Scan Meditation: Body scan meditation is another mindfulness practice that systematically directs attention to different body parts. This practice enhances somatic awareness, allowing individuals to observe the subtle sensations and energy movements associated with Kundalini awakening. The body scan becomes a tool for exploring the intricate connection between the physical body and energy flow, promoting a holistic understanding of the awakening process.

Non-Judgmental Awareness: Mindfulness during Kundalini awakening emphasizes non-judgmental awareness, encouraging individuals to release habitual patterns of self-criticism or judgment. As Kundalini energy activates and purifies various aspects of the being, individuals may encounter aspects of themselves that elicit discomfort or resistance. A non-judgmental attitude allows for self-acceptance, acknowledging each experience as a natural and integral part of the awakening journey.

Integrating Mindfulness into Daily Life: Cultivating mindfulness is not confined to formal meditation sessions; it extends into daily life. Individuals are encouraged to bring mindful awareness to routine activities, interactions, and challenges. This integration supports the continuity of self-awareness, allowing individuals to embody mindfulness in all aspects of their existence. The fluid integration of mindfulness into daily life serves as a bridge between meditative insights and the practical realities of navigating the awakened state.

Self-Inquiry: Mindfulness during Kundalini awakening often involves self-inquiry—an introspective exploration of the nature of the self, identity, and the underlying motivations of thought and behavior. They engage in self-inquiry, which prompts individuals to question deeply ingrained beliefs and assumptions, fostering a profound understanding of the self beyond the egoic mind. This process of inquiry aligns with the transformative potential of Kundalini awakening, encouraging a radical shift in one's sense of identity and self-perception.

Acceptance of the Present Moment: Mindfulness inherently involves the acceptance of the present moment, acknowledging it as it is without the desire for it to be different. This acceptance becomes particularly relevant during Kundalini awakening, where individuals may encounter a spectrum of experiences—joyful, challenging, or ethereal. Acceptance does not imply passive resignation but rather embracing each moment with an open heart and a receptive mind. This attitude fosters resilience and adaptability, qualities crucial for navigating the diverse terrain of Kundalini activation.

Awareness of Energetic Shifts: Mindfulness during Kundalini awakening extends to the awareness of energetic shifts within the body. Sensations of warmth, tingling, or the movement of energy along the spine become objects of attention during mindfulness practices. By directing focused awareness to these subtle, energetic phenomena, individuals deepen their connection to the unfolding Kundalini process. This heightened sensitivity to the active body contributes to a more nuanced and embodied understanding of the awakening journey.

Mindful Integration of Spiritual Insights: Kundalini awakening often brings forth profound spiritual insights and expanded states of consciousness. Mindfulness facilitates the integration of these insights into daily life, ensuring that the transformative revelations do not remain confined to meditative experiences but permeate the fabric of one's existence. Mindful integration supports individuals in embodying the wisdom gained during heightened awareness, fostering a harmonious alignment between the spiritual and material aspects of life.

Guidance and Support: While mindfulness provides a valuable framework for self-awareness during Kundalini awakening, seeking guidance from experienced mentors or teachers is equally important. Knowledgeable guides can offer insights, reassurance, and practical advice based on their experiences with Kundalini energy. This external support complements the internal journey of self-awareness, creating a balanced approach that combines personal exploration with the wisdom of those who have traversed similar paths.

In conclusion, cultivating mindfulness and self-awareness during Kundalini awakening is a transformative practice that aligns the individual with the unfolding journey of spiritual awakening. Mindfulness becomes a guiding light, illuminating the intricate landscape of thoughts, emotions, and energetic shifts. This intentional presence fosters a deepened understanding of the self and the profound potential inherent in Kundalini activation. As individuals navigate the challenges and revelations of this awakening process, mindfulness serves as a steady companion, offering a grounded and compassionate awareness that supports the harmonious integration of the awakened state into daily life.

Creating a supportive environment for the awakening process

Establishing a nurturing atmosphere is essential for promoting the Kundalini awakening process. The transformation road entails reawakening the latent spiritual force at the spine's base. Kundalini's awakening energy and spiritual aspects require a supportive external environment that balances the internal changes and difficulties people may experience. A supportive environment has several facets, such as relationships, physical space, and lifestyle choices, all essential to creating a peaceful, secure setting in which the Kundalini journey can emerge.

Physical Space: Establishing a serene and energetically balanced physical space is fundamental for individuals undergoing Kundalini awakening. A clutter-free, clean environment with ample natural light fosters a sense of tranquility and promotes overall well-being. Creating a dedicated meditation space within the home allows individuals to cultivate a consistent practice and encourages a connection with the divine during moments of stillness. The vibrational quality of the physical surroundings influences the energetic body, and a consciously arranged space can enhance the flow of Kundalini energy.

Nature Connection: Engaging with nature is integral to creating a supportive environment for Kundalini awakening. Spending time outdoors, whether in a garden, park, or natural setting, allows individuals to connect with the earth's grounding energy. Nature serves as a mirror for the transformative processes occurring within, offering solace, inspiration, and a reminder of the interconnectedness of all life. Regular walks in nature, contemplation under the open sky, and connecting with the natural elements contribute to a balanced and harmonious external environment.

Relationships and Community: Building supportive relationships is essential during the Kundalini awakening process. They share experiences with like-minded individuals through spiritual communities, workshops, or online forums, which provides a sense of connection and validation. Engaging with a supportive community allows for exchanging insights, encouragement, and guidance, reducing feelings of isolation that may arise during the transformative journey. Cultivating open communication with friends and family members, even if they do not share the same spiritual perspectives, fosters understanding and emotional support.

Energetic Hygiene: Maintaining energetic hygiene is vital in creating a supportive environment for Kundalini awakening. Practices such as smudging with sage or other purifying herbs, using crystals, and engaging in energy-clearing rituals help to cleanse the energetic space. Regularly clearing the energy within the home, especially the meditation space, ensures that it remains conducive to the flow of Kundalini energy. Energetic hygiene extends to personal practices, encouraging individuals to be mindful of their energetic boundaries and engage in practices that promote energetic balance.

Nutrition and Lifestyle: Adopting a balanced and nourishing lifestyle contributes to the supportive environment necessary for Kundalini awakening. Nutrition is crucial, emphasizing a plant-based, whole-food diet that enhances physical vitality and energetic balance. Adequate hydration supports the body's detoxification processes, aiding in the purification associated with Kundalini activation. Regular exercise, yoga, or other mindful movement practices promote overall well-being and facilitate the smooth flow of energy within the body.

Mindful Media Consumption: Awareness of media consumption creates a supportive environment for Kundalini awakening. Limiting exposure to harmful or overly stimulating content, including news, movies, or social media, helps maintain a focused and centered mental state. Choosing media that aligns with spiritual or uplifting themes contributes to a positive and harmonious mental environment. A conscious and discerning approach to media consumption supports cultivating a clear and receptive mind during the awakening process.

Sacred Rituals and Practices: Incorporating holy rituals and practices into daily life enhances the supportive environment for Kundalini awakening. This may include morning rituals, prayer, or meditation sessions that set the tone for the day. Creating a sense of sacredness in everyday activities, such as cooking, bathing, or walking, elevates the vibrational frequency of these experiences. Rituals provide a framework for intentional living, anchoring individuals in a spiritually attuned mindset throughout their daily routines.

Educational Resources: Establishing a conducive atmosphere for Kundalini awakening requires having access to advice and educational materials. Knowledge and essential insights about Kundalini energy and spiritual awakening can be gained through reading books, attending seminars, or taking online courses. Knowing the many phases of the Kundalini process, possible obstacles, and valuable techniques enables people to proceed with awareness and discernment on their path. Seeking advice from knowledgeable mentors or instructors further strengthens the supportive environment's educational component.

Recognizing that the journey is highly individualized and may unfold unexpectedly allows individuals to approach challenges with resilience and an open heart. Embracing change and remaining receptive to the guidance of the Kundalini energy promotes a fluid and harmonious relationship with the transformative forces at play.

In conclusion, creating a supportive environment for Kundalini awakening involves a holistic approach that addresses physical, emotional, and energetic dimensions. The external setting becomes a mirror for the internal journey, offering a foundation of stability, nourishment, and inspiration. The synergy of a harmonious physical space, meaningful relationships, mindful lifestyle choices, and a commitment to spiritual practices creates an environment that encourages the safe and transformative unfolding of the Kundalini awakening process. As individuals cultivate a supportive external environment, they simultaneously nurture the inner landscape, fostering a profound connection to the divine and the expansive realms of consciousness.

CHAPTER V

Kundalini Yoga and Meditation Techniques

Introduction to Kundalini yoga

This style of yoga, which has its roots in the idea of Kundalini energy—characterized as a coiled serpent at the base of the spine—aims to awaken and harness this latent spiritual potential through dynamic postures, breathing exercises, meditation, and chanting. The three main goals of Kundalini yoga are expanding awareness, releasing spiritual potential, and cultivating a strong bond between the person and the global life force.

At the heart of Kundalini Yoga is the belief that each person possesses a dormant reserve of vital energy coiled at the base of the spine, often depicted metaphorically as a serpent. This stagnant energy, known as Kundalini, is the potential source of spiritual enlightenment and self-realization. Kundalini Yoga aims to activate and guide this energy upward through the central energy channel, aligning and balancing the various energy centers, or chakras, along the spine.

A distinctive feature of Kundalini Yoga is its emphasis on combining physical postures (asanas), breath control (pranayama), and chanting (mantra) in a cohesive and dynamic sequence. The practice is designed to work simultaneously on multiple levels—physical, mental, and energetic—. The asanas engage the body and enhance flexibility, strength, and balance. The pranayama techniques regulate the breath, increasing the flow of life force energy throughout the body. Chanting mantras, often accompanied by specific hand gestures (mudras), stimulate the vibrational frequencies within the body, aligning the practitioner with higher states of consciousness.

The Kundalini Yoga tradition is attributed to Yogi Bhajan, who introduced this ancient practice to the West in the late 1960s. Yogi Bhajan emphasized the accessibility of Kundalini Yoga, presenting it as a practical and transformative tool for individuals seeking spiritual growth in the modern world. The core tenet of Yogi Bhajan's teachings is that everyone is born with the ability to encounter the divine within, and Kundalini Yoga offers a systematic way to awaken this potential.

This is a characteristic that sets the classes apart. This chant sets the tone for the practice by creating a sacred space and connecting the practitioner to the lineage of teachers who have transmitted this wisdom throughout millennia. In class, a kriya (a blend of breathing exercises, postures, and meditation techniques) is usually worked through to address a specific aspect of the self or to achieve a particular objective.

The practice of breathwork, or pranayama, is essential to Kundalini Yoga. Prana, or life force energy, can be controlled and directed using techniques like Breath of Fire, a fast and rhythmic breathing technique, and Nadi Shodhana, an alternative nostril breathing technique. Conscious, regulated breathing is one of the most powerful strategies for bringing Kundalini energy to life and achieving heightened awareness.

Meditation is an integral component of Kundalini Yoga, and each kriya concludes with a period of deep meditation. Practitioners may be guided through specific meditations, focusing on breath awareness, mantra repetition, or visualization. The meditative aspect of Kundalini Yoga aims to quiet the mind, expand consciousness, and create a profound connection to the divine.

Chanting mantras is a distinctive and potent element of Kundalini Yoga. Mantras are sacred sound vibrations that carry specific frequencies and meanings. The vibrational quality of mantras stimulates the chakras, balances the nervous system, and elevates the practitioner's consciousness. The chanting of mantras is often accompanied by specific hand movements or mudras, further enhancing the energetic impact of the practice.

Kundalini Yoga significantly affects the practitioner's energetic and spiritual aspects and the physical and cerebral domains. A more vital link to the universal life force, elevated states of awareness, and expanded consciousness are thought to result from the awakening of Kundalini energy. The practice is open to people of many origins and faiths because it is not restricted to any particular religion or philosophy.

Kundalini Yoga is considered a holistic science that integrates various yogic tools to bring about a holistic transformation. It is designed to awaken the dormant potential within each individual, encouraging self-discovery and spiritual evolution. As the Kundalini energy rises through the spine, it purifies and balances the chakras, leading to a harmonious integration of the self's physical, mental, and spiritual aspects.

In conclusion, Kundalini Yoga is a unique and transformative path within the rich tapestry of yogic traditions. Its dynamic and multifaceted approach, combining physical postures, breathwork, chanting, and meditation, offers practitioners a comprehensive toolkit for self-discovery and spiritual growth. Rooted in ancient wisdom yet accessible to modern seekers, Kundalini Yoga continues to inspire individuals on their journey towards expanded consciousness, inner awakening, and a profound connection to the divine.

Specific yoga poses and meditation techniques for Kundalini awakening

The Kundalini awakening journey takes a systematic and deliberate approach to awaken the latent spiritual energy coiling at the base of the spine. Certain yoga poses and meditation practices are integral to the rich tapestry of Kundalini Yoga; they aid in the upward flow of Kundalini energy, cleanse the energy centers, or chakras, and promote a harmonious union of the mind, body, and spirit. These practices are carefully curated to activate and balance the subtle energy channels, creating a conducive environment for the transformative journey of Kundalini awakening. Yoga Poses for Kundalini Awakening:

Serpent Pose (Bhujangasana): This backbend posture, often called the Cobra Pose, activates the lower spine and stimulates the sacral and root chakras. Bhujangasana opens the heart center, promoting a sense of expansion and receptivity to the upward movement of Kundalini energy.

Camel Pose (Ustrasana): Ustrasana is a deep backbend that targets the throat and heart chakras. The expansive nature of this pose facilitates the flow of energy through the upper body, encouraging the awakening of higher centers and promoting a sense of openness and surrender.

Bow Pose (Dhanurasana): Dhanurasana is a dynamic backbend that engages the entire spine. This pose stimulates the solar plexus chakra, promoting personal power and will activation. The back arching creates a mighty stretch, releasing tension and energetic blockages.

Root Lock (Mulabandha): While not a traditional yoga pose, Mulabandha is a yogic lock that involves engaging the pelvic floor muscles. This energetic lock directs the flow of Kundalini energy upward, preventing it from dissipating and ensuring its concentrated ascent through the central energy channel.

Shoulder Stand (Sarvangasana): Sarvangasana, or Shoulder Stand, is an inversion that directs energy toward the throat chakra. In this pose, the body is supported on the shoulders, and the throat is open, creating a pathway for the upward movement of Kundalini energy.

Crow Pose (Bakasana): Bakasana, or Crow Pose, is an arm balance that activates the lower chakras and promotes grounding. The focused engagement required in this pose builds strength and stability, creating a foundation for the safe ascent of Kundalini energy.

The Eagle Pose, also known as Garudasana, is a balancing pose in which you cross one leg over the other and cross your arms. This pose promotes the body's natural flow of energy by igniting the energy centers in the arms and legs.

Meditation Techniques for Kundalini Awakening:

Kirtan Kriya: Kirtan Kriya is a chanting meditation involving the repetition of the mantra "Sa Ta Na Ma." As each syllable is chanted, specific finger movements (mudras) accompany the sounds. This meditation technique activates the brain centers, harmonizes the chakras, and facilitates the upward movement of Kundalini energy.

Third Eye Meditation: One of the most effective meditation techniques for Kundalini awakening is focusing attention on the area between the eyebrows, sometimes known as the ajna chakra or third eye. By focusing inward, practitioners can reach heightened awareness and activate the energy center linked to spiritual insight and intuition.

Chakra Meditation: Chakra meditation sequentially focuses on the seven main chakras, starting from the root and ascending to the crown. This meditation technique brings awareness to each energy center, promoting balance, alignment, and the free flow of Kundalini energy through subtle channels.

Breath of Fire Meditation: Breath of Fire is a rapid and rhythmic breathwork technique involving quick, active nose breathing. This dynamic meditation technique oxygenates the body, energizes the nervous system, and activates the solar plexus chakra, promoting the awakening of personal power.

Sitali Pranayama: Sitali Pranayama, or cooling breath, involves inhaling through a curled tongue and exhaling through the nose. This breathwork technique balances the body's temperature, purifies the bloodstream, and activates the throat chakra, creating a conducive environment for the ascent of Kundalini energy.

Navel Center Meditation: Focusing on the navel center, or manipura chakra, brings attention to the area associated with personal power and transformation. This meditation technique involves visualizing a radiant sun at the navel, encouraging the activation of the solar plexus chakra and facilitating the upward movement of Kundalini energy.

Silent Witness Meditation: Silent Witness Meditation involves cultivating the role of the silent observer, witnessing thoughts, emotions, and sensations without attachment. By detaching from the fluctuations of the mind, practitioners create a spacious internal environment, allowing for the unimpeded flow of Kundalini energy.

Integration of Yoga Poses and Meditation:

The synergy of specific yoga poses and meditation techniques creates a holistic approach to Kundalini awakening. Yoga poses prepare the physical body by stretching, strengthening, and balancing, while meditation techniques focus the mind and direct energy toward specific chakras. The combined practice cultivates a receptive and harmonious internal environment, facilitating the smooth ascent of Kundalini energy through subtle channels.

It is crucial to approach these practices with mindfulness, patience, and a deep connection to one's inner wisdom. Kundalini awakening is a highly individualized process, and each practitioner may respond differently to various poses and meditation techniques. Seeking guidance from experienced teachers or mentors familiar with Kundalini Yoga ensures that individuals embark on this transformative journey with the necessary support and insights.

In conclusion, the specific yoga poses and meditation techniques within the realm of Kundalini Yoga provide a structured and potent framework for awakening dormant spiritual energy. Through the intentional combination of dynamic postures, breathwork, and focused meditation, practitioners create an internal landscape conducive to the safe and transformative ascent of Kundalini energy. As individuals engage in these practices with reverence and awareness, they open themselves to the profound potential for expanded consciousness, self-realization, and a deepened connection to the universal life force.

Breathwork and including visualization exercises

Breathwork and visualization exercises are essential to Kundalini Yoga, leading practitioners on a profound journey of self-discovery and spiritual awakening. These ancient yoga techniques, rooted in wisdom from the yogic tradition, use the breath and the power of the mind to awaken dormant energy, balance the chakras, and encourage the upward movement of Kundalini, the coiled serpent of spiritual potential at the base of the spine. Pranayama, breathing exercises, and visualization techniques combine to produce a transforming and harmonious interior environment that opens the door to increased awareness and a stronger connection to the universal life force.

Breath of Fire (Agni Pran): A hallmark of Kundalini Yoga, Breath of Fire is a rapid and rhythmic breath that involves pumping the navel point with each exhale and allowing the inhale to happen naturally. This dynamic breathwork technique oxygenates the body, energizes the nervous system, and stokes the internal fire. Breath of Fire is believed to stimulate the solar plexus chakra, fostering the awakening of personal power and vitality.

Long, Deep Breathing (Dirgha Pranayama): This breathwork technique involves slow, deep inhalations and exhalations through the nose. Deep Breathing calms the nervous system, balances the flow of prana (life force energy), and activates the heart center. As practitioners cultivate a conscious and deliberate breath, they create a foundation for the smooth and controlled movement of Kundalini energy through the central energy channel.

Alternate Nostril Breathing (Nadi Shodhana): Nadi Shodhana is a balancing breathwork technique that involves alternating between the nostrils using the fingers to regulate the flow of breath. This practice harmonizes the left and right energy channels, promoting balance within the body and mind. Nadi Shodhana activates the third eye and crown chakras, fostering clarity and expanded consciousness.

Breath Retention (Kumbhaka): Incorporating periods of breath retention, or Kumbhaka, into the breathwork practice is common in Kundalini Yoga. After a deep inhalation, practitioners may retain the breath, allowing the energy to circulate and accumulate before exhaling. Kumbhaka enhances the capacity to harness and direct prana, creating a reservoir of vital energy for the awakening of Kundalini.

Chakra Visualization: Practitioners frequently employ chakra visualization exercises to focus attention and energy on specific energy centers along the spine. Chakras can be more easily purified and activated by visualizing each one as a spinning wheel of light that starts at the root and moves up to the crown. This exercise corresponds with the chakra system's upward flow of Kundalini energy.

Golden Cord Meditation: In this visualization, practitioners imagine a golden cord extending from the spine's base to the head's crown. This cord represents the central energy channel, also known as the Sushumna. By visualizing energy flow along this golden cord, individuals enhance their awareness of Kundalini's ascent and foster a connection to the divine.

Lotus Flower Meditation: Lotus Flower Meditation involves visualizing a lotus flower at each chakra, with each flower unfolding and blooming as the corresponding energy center is activated. This practice symbolizes the blossoming of consciousness and the transformative journey of Kundalini's awakening. The imagery of the lotus aligns with spiritual purity and enlightenment.

Third Eye Activation: Visualization exercises often focus on the third eye, located between the eyebrows. Practitioners may visualize a radiant light or a specific symbol, such as an Om or a lotus, at the third eye center. This practice stimulates the ajna chakra, promoting intuition, insight, and the expansion of consciousness—a crucial aspect of Kundalini awakening.

Serpentine Visualization: Given the serpent metaphor associated with Kundalini, practitioners may visualize a serpent coiled at the base of the spine. As the breath and energy rise, the serpent gradually uncoils and ascends through the central energy channel, symbolizing the awakening and ascent of Kundalini energy. This visualization aligns with the transformative process of shedding old layers and embracing higher states of consciousness.

Combining breathwork and visualization in Kundalini Yoga creates a dynamic and potent synergy. As practitioners engage in specific breathwork techniques, they synchronize the breath with visualizations that direct energy and awareness to critical aspects of the subtle body. The breath becomes a vehicle for the flow of prana, while the mind's eye directs and amplifies the energetic focus. As a result of this harmonic connection, one's consciousness is raised, which facilitates the safe and transformational ascent of Kundalini energy.

The relationship between visualization and breathwork creates a link between the practice's energy and physical aspects. Prana is carried by breath, and the conscious direction of that life force is guided by visualization. This purposeful connection creates a holistic approach to Kundalini's awakening by addressing the subtle and physiological parts of the practitioner's existence.

While breathwork and visualization are powerful tools in Kundalini Yoga, it is essential to approach these practices with mindfulness and respect for individual experiences. Kundalini awakening is a highly personal journey, and practitioners may encounter intense sensations, emotional releases, or heightened states of awareness.

Seeking guidance from experienced teachers and practicing under their supervision ensures a supportive and informed approach to these transformative techniques.

In conclusion, breathwork and visualization exercises in Kundalini Yoga form an inseparable duo that guides practitioners on a transformative journey toward self-realization. As individuals harness the power of the breath and engage the creative potential of the mind's eye, they create a dynamic synergy that aligns with the profound Kundalini awakening process. The intentional integration of breath and visualization enhances the practice. It serves as a gateway to expanded consciousness, spiritual insight, and a deepened connection to the inherent wisdom of the self.

CHAPTER VI

The Role of Energy Healing

Exploring various energy healing modalities

In the expansive realm of holistic wellness, diverse energy healing modalities have emerged, each offering unique approaches to promote balance, harmony, and well-being on physical, emotional, and spiritual levels. These modalities are founded on the principle that the body possesses an intricate energy system that can be influenced and balanced to support optimal health. By acknowledging the interconnectedness of the mind, body, and energy, practitioners of energy healing modalities aim to restore and enhance the flow of vital life force energy. This section explores some prominent energy healing modalities, delving into their principles, techniques, and potential benefits.

Reiki is a Japanese energy healing method that promotes healing and balance by channelling universal life force energy. Reiki practitioners attuned to the symbols transfer this energy to the recipient, who may be lying down, sitting, or fully dressed. The gentle touch or hands-hovering technique facilitates the healing energy, which treats physical illnesses and mental imbalances and promotes relaxation. Reiki is frequently described as relaxing; people who get it report feeling warm, tingly, and profoundly relaxed during and after sessions.

The goal is to maintain equilibrium in the flow of Qi, the life force that keeps the body alive. Acupuncture treats imbalances eases pain, and promotes general well-being by increasing or decreasing energy flow at particular locations. The method is acknowledged for its efficacy in treating a range of medical disorders, including chronic pain, stress, and other ailments.

They are derived from ancient Indian spiritual traditions; chakra healing centers around the body's seven energy centers, or chakras. These spinning wheels of energy are associated with different physical, emotional, and spiritual well-being aspects. Various techniques, including meditation, visualization, and energy work, balance and activate the chakras. Practitioners believe harmonizing the chakras promotes a free energy flow throughout the body, fostering holistic health and supporting spiritual development.

The energy qualities of crystals and gemstones are used in crystal therapy to bring harmony and balance back to the body's energy field. Specific crystals are thought to resonate with particular energy centres; therefore, during sessions, practitioners may lay crystals on or near the body. It is believed that the distinct vibrational frequencies of the crystals affect the flow of energy, clearing obstructions and fostering healing. Crystal healing is frequently combined with other energy therapies to provide a holistic approach to health.

Pranic Healing, developed by Master Choa Kok Sui, is based on the concept of prana, the vital life force energy that sustains the body. Practitioners employ techniques to cleanse, energize, and balance the body's energy field. Pranic Healing involves scanning the energy body, removing congested or depleted energy, and infusing fresh, vital energy to facilitate healing. This non-touch modality is utilized for various physical and emotional ailments, emphasizing the importance of maintaining a balanced energy system for overall health.

Quantum healing is grounded in the principles of quantum physics and the interconnectedness of energy and matter. Practitioners in quantum healing work with the idea that shifts in the energetic and vibrational aspects of the body can influence physical and emotional well-being. Techniques may include visualization, intention setting, and energy clearing to create a quantum shift in the individual's energy field. Quantum healing acknowledges the inherent relationship between consciousness and energy, suggesting that changes in one aspect can influence the other.

Sound healing utilizes the vibrational frequencies of sound to restore balance and promote healing. Instruments such as Tibetan singing bowls, tuning forks, and gongs create resonant frequencies interacting with the body's energy field. The vibrations dissolve energetic blockages, stimulate energy flow, and induce deep relaxation. Sound healing is versatile, with practices ranging from individual sessions to group experiences, where the collective vibration contributes to a harmonious energy exchange.

Energy psychology encompasses modalities like the Emotional Freedom Technique (EFT) and Thought Field Therapy (TFT). These approaches combine psychological principles with understanding the body's energy system. By tapping on specific acupressure points or using other techniques, practitioners aim to release emotional blockages and rewire negative thought patterns. Energy psychology recognizes the link between emotions, thoughts, and energy, offering a holistic mental and emotional well-being approach.

Rooted in ancient indigenous practices, shamanic healing involves the practitioner entering altered states of consciousness to connect with spiritual realms for guidance and healing. Various techniques, such as journeying, soul retrieval, and energy extraction, are employed to address spiritual imbalances and energetic intrusions and facilitate the integration of lost or fragmented aspects of the self. Shamanic healing recognizes the importance of the spiritual dimension in overall well-being.

Investigating different energy healing treatments exposes the wide range of strategies that promote harmony, balance, and well-being. Each modality has its own beliefs and methods. Still, they all share an understanding of the body's subtle energy system and how it significantly affects mental, emotional, and spiritual well-being. Integrating energy healing techniques offers a holistic and complementary approach to traditional healthcare as people traverse their wellness journeys, encouraging a better knowledge of the interconnectedness between energy, consciousness, and vibrant well-being.

How energy healing can aid in Kundalini activation

The ancient practice of Kundalini Yoga, rooted in the profound wisdom of the yogic tradition, unveils the transformative potential of dormant spiritual energy coiled at the base of the spine. Known as Kundalini, this potent force is believed to carry the power of self- realization and spiritual enlightenment. While the journey of Kundalini activation is profoundly personal and requires dedicated practice, incorporating energy healing modalities can offer invaluable support in facilitating a smooth and harmonious awakening. Energy healing, focusing on balancing and enhancing the flow of vital life force energy, aligns seamlessly with the principles of Kundalini Yoga, creating a synergistic approach to spiritual evolution.

Reiki, a Japanese energy healing technique, stands out as a modality that complements the process of Kundalini activation. Reiki practitioners, attuned to the universal life force energy, act as conduits for channeling this energy to the recipient. The gentle touch or hands-hovering technique in Reiki aligns with the subtlety required in Kundalini activation, where the practitioner seeks to awaken the dormant energy within. The calming effect of Reiki promotes relaxation, which is conducive to the safe ascent of Kundalini energy. Recipients often report sensations of warmth, tingling, and profound peace during Reiki sessions, providing a harmonious environment for the transformative Kundalini journey.

Acupuncture, rooted in Traditional Chinese Medicine, offers another avenue for supporting Kundalini activation through energy healing. Acupuncture is a Chinese medicine that balances the flow of Qi, or life force energy, by carefully placing tiny needles into specific places throughout the body's meridians. Acupuncture helps to harmonize energy channels inside the Kundalini system, where the ascent of energy is a focus point. Acupuncture facilitates the free passage of energy by treating potential obstructions or imbalances in the meridians. This creates an atmosphere favorable for Kundalini to rise through the Sushumna, the primary energy channel.

Chakra healing, deeply intertwined with Kundalini Yoga philosophy, emphasizes the balanced functioning of the body's energy centers. The chakras, spinning wheels of energy aligned along the spine, play a crucial role in the Kundalini activation process. Energy healing modalities focusing on chakra alignments, such as meditation, visualization, and energy work, contribute to the purification and activation of these energy centers. By ensuring that the chakras are open and balanced, energy healing facilitates the smooth flow of Kundalini energy through subtle channels, fostering holistic well-being and spiritual growth.

Crystal healing, leveraging the vibrational frequencies of crystals and gemstones, aligns with the energetic principles of Kundalini activation. Crystals are believed to resonate with specific energy centers, making them valuable tools in balancing and awakening Kundalini. Practitioners may place crystals on or around the body, harnessing their unique properties to clear energetic blockages and enhance the flow of Kundalini energy.

Intentionally using crystals in energy healing sessions creates a supportive and highly vibrant environment conducive to Kundalini's transformative journey.

Pranic Healing, a modality developed by Master Choa Kok Sui, offers targeted techniques to cleanse, energize, and balance the body's energy field. The emphasis on prana, the vital life force energy, resonates with the core principle of Kundalini activation. Pranic Healing involves scanning the energy body, removing congested or depleted energy, and infusing fresh, vital energy to facilitate healing. This non-touch modality aligns with the subtlety required in Kundalini's work, where the practitioner aims to promote the upward movement of energy with precision and care.

Quantum healing, drawing inspiration from the principles of quantum physics, expands the understanding of how energy healing can aid in Kundalini activation. Quantum healing recognizes the interconnectedness of energy and consciousness, suggesting that shifts in one aspect can influence the other. Techniques involving visualization, intention setting, and energy clearing create a quantum change in the individual's energy field. This resonates with the transformative nature of Kundalini activation, where shifts in consciousness and energy are interwoven in the journey towards self-realization.

Sound healing, with its emphasis on the vibrational frequencies of sound, provides an additional dimension to energy healing in the context of Kundalini activation. Instruments such as Tibetan singing bowls, tuning forks, and gongs produce resonant frequencies interacting with the body's energy field. The vibrations dissolve energetic blockages, stimulate energy flow, and induce deep relaxation. Sound healing aligns with the ancient wisdom of Kundalini Yoga, where mantras, chants, and sounds play a significant role in awakening and harmonizing the dormant spiritual energy.

Energy psychology, encompassing modalities like the Emotional Freedom Technique (EFT) and Thought Field Therapy (TFT), bridges the gap between psychology and energy work in Kundalini activation. These approaches combine psychological principles with understanding the body's energy system. By tapping on specific acupressure points or using other techniques, energy psychology aims to release emotional blockages and rewire negative thought patterns. This integration recognizes the intimate connection between emotions, thoughts, and energy—essential considerations in the Kundalini awakening process.

Shamanic healing, deeply rooted in ancient indigenous practices, contributes a spiritual dimension to the energy healing landscape that resonates with Kundalini activation. Shamanic techniques, such as journeying, soul retrieval, and energy extraction, address spiritual imbalances and facilitate the integration of lost or fragmented aspects of the self. The shamanic perspective acknowledges the importance of the spiritual dimension in the overall well-being of an individual—a fundamental element of Kundalini activation.

In conclusion, integrating energy healing modalities can significantly aid Kundalini activation, providing valuable support for individuals on their spiritual journey. These modalities, each with unique principles and techniques, create a holistic and complementary approach to Kundalini Yoga. The harmonization, balancing, and elevation of vital life force energy fostered by energy healing align seamlessly with the transformative journey of Kundalini awakening, contributing to the evolution of consciousness, self-realization, and the deepening connection to the universal life force. As practitioners navigate the path of Kundalini activation, the synergy between energy healing and ancient yogic wisdom illuminates a path of profound spiritual growth and self-discovery.

Working with healers and practitioners

Embarking on a journey of holistic wellness often involves seeking guidance and support from healers and practitioners who specialize in various modalities. The collaboration between individuals on their wellness journey and experienced healers creates a dynamic relationship that can significantly impact physical, emotional, and spiritual well-being. Whether navigating specific health challenges, exploring personal growth, or delving into spiritual practices, the synergy between seekers and healers forms a crucial aspect of the holistic healing process.

Energy healing practitioners are pivotal in supporting individuals seeking to balance and harmonize their energetic bodies. Modalities such as Reiki, Pranic Healing, and Chakra Balancing involve manipulating and enhancing the subtle energy that flows through the body. When working with energy healers, individuals often experience a deep sense of relaxation and a release of energetic blockages. The practitioner serves as a conduit for channeling universal life force energy, removing stagnant energy, and promoting a free flow of vitality. Individuals can actively engage in their healing process through the collaborative aspect of energy healing sessions, which fosters a sense of empowerment and a connection to one's life force.

In addition, traditional medicine practitioners—such as physicians, nurses, and other medical specialists—are essential to pursuing holistic well-being. Integrative medicine methods acknowledge the benefits of complementary and alternative therapeutic therapies in addition to traditional medical procedures. Collaborating with conventional medicine practitioners ensures a thorough grasp of a person's health and well-being. People can develop a comprehensive strategy that considers their health's physical and energetic facets by exchanging insights about holistic practices. A collaborative and well-informed decision-making process is facilitated by open and transparent communication and transparency between patients and healthcare providers.

Holistic counselors and therapists offer support on the emotional and psychological fronts, addressing the interconnected nature of mental and physical health. Modalities such as psychotherapy, counseling, and mindfulness-based therapies provide individuals with tools to navigate challenges, process emotions, and cultivate resilience. The therapeutic relationship fosters a safe space for individuals to explore the root causes of emotional imbalances and develop coping strategies. Collaborating with holistic counselors allows individuals to gain insights into the mind-body connection, creating a foundation for comprehensive well-being.

Nutritionists and dieticians are crucial in guiding individuals toward optimal physical health through personalized dietary plans. The importance of nutrition in holistic wellness cannot be overstated, as the food we consume directly influences our energy levels, mental clarity, and overall vitality. Collaborating with nutrition professionals allows individuals to tailor their diets to support their unique health needs. Integrating nutritional guidance with other healing modalities ensures a holistic approach to well-being, addressing the body's physical requirements in conjunction with energy and emotional balance.

For those on a spiritual journey, seeking guidance from spiritual guides and mentors can provide invaluable support. These individuals often deeply understand spiritual practices, meditation, and ancient wisdom traditions. Whether exploring Kundalini awakening, meditation techniques or connecting with higher states of consciousness, spiritual guides offer insights and techniques to facilitate personal growth and self-realization. Along the spiritual path, the mentor-mentee connection provides support and direction by fostering community and shared discovery.

Bodywork and movement practitioners, including massage therapists, yoga instructors, and somatic practitioners, contribute to holistic wellness by addressing the physical body. Bodywork modalities release tension, improve circulation, and support the body's natural healing processes. Collaborating with these practitioners enhances the overall sense of well-being, promoting flexibility, relaxation, and alignment. Through therapeutic massage, yoga, or somatic movement practices, individuals can actively care for and maintain their physical bodies, complementing other aspects of their holistic wellness journey.

Mind-body practitioners—including those specializing in mindfulness, meditation, and breathwork—offer strategies for developing emotional stability, mental clarity, and inner calm. Working with these practitioners enables people to create mindfulness practices that suit their requirements and objectives. Methods such as mindfulness meditation help people feel less stressed, focus better, and have better emotional health. People can incorporate these techniques into their daily lives with the support of mind-body practitioners, creating a long-lasting basis for holistic wellness.

Herbalists and alternative medicine practitioners offer insights into natural remedies and plant-based therapies that can support overall health. Herbal medicine, traditional healing practices, and alternative therapies can complement conventional medical approaches. Collaborating with herbalists allows individuals to explore the benefits of botanical remedies, dietary supplements, and holistic approaches to wellness. Integrating alternative medicine with other healing modalities offers a diverse and personalized approach to holistic well- being.

In navigating the collaborative process with healers and practitioners, individuals are encouraged to approach each interaction with an open mind and clear communication. Establishing trust and rapport with these professionals fosters a supportive environment for holistic healing. To guarantee a customized and all-encompassing approach, people must actively participate in their treatment process by communicating their experiences, worries, and objectives to practitioners. A potent synergy that recognizes the complex nature of holistic wellness is produced when seekers and healers work together, opening the door to transformative and long-lasting well-being.

CHAPTER VII

Challenges and Solutions

Common obstacles faced during Kundalini awakening

The journey of Kundalini awakening, a profound spiritual transformation and self-realization process, is not without its challenges. As individuals navigate the intricate pathways of energy ascent and heightened consciousness, they may encounter various obstacles that test their resolve and understanding. Recognizing and understanding these common obstacles is crucial for those on the Kundalini path, as it allows for informed and empowered navigation through the ups and downs of this transformative journey.

Intensity of Energy: One of the primary obstacles faced during Kundalini awakening is the intensity of energy accompanying the rising Kundalini. As this potent energy ascends through the central energy channel, known as the Sushumna, individuals may experience overwhelming sensations, energy surges, and heightened states of awareness. The intensity can be challenging to integrate into daily life, leading to feelings of disorientation or even physical discomfort. Practitioners must cultivate practices that ground and stabilize their energy, such as mindful breathing, gentle movement, and spending time in nature.

Emotional Release: Kundalini's awakening often triggers a profound release of stored emotions, memories, and unresolved experiences. This emotional release can manifest as intense mood swings, heightened sensitivity, or even periods of emotional turbulence. Individuals may confront past traumas or face deep-seated fears during this process. The challenge lies in navigating these emotional currents with self-compassion and understanding. Integrating therapeutic practices, such as journaling, counseling, or engaging in creative expression, can provide a constructive outlet for processing and releasing these emotions.

Physical Discomfort: The activation of Kundalini energy can have tangible effects on the physical body, ranging from mild discomfort to more pronounced sensations. Practitioners may experience muscle cramps, involuntary movements, or heat or cold sensations. These physical manifestations can be disconcerting, and individuals may question whether these sensations indicate a health concern. Seeking guidance from holistic healthcare practitioners who understand Kundalini dynamics can help individuals differentiate between normal energetic sensations and potential health issues, providing reassurance and appropriate support.

Disruption of Daily Life: Kundalini awakening is a transformative process that can disrupt established routines and patterns. As individuals undergo shifts in consciousness and energy, they may find it challenging to maintain a sense of normalcy in their daily lives. Relationships, work, and social dynamics may be influenced, leading to a period of adjustment. Balancing the demands of daily responsibilities with the inward focus required for Kundalini activation poses a common challenge. Integrating mindfulness practices, time management strategies, and communication with loved ones can help individuals navigate this transition period.

Unsettling Psychic Experiences: As Kundalini energy activates higher states of consciousness, individuals may encounter psychic experiences that challenge their understanding of reality. These experiences can include vivid dreams, heightened intuition, or even glimpses into expanded states of awareness. While these psychic phenomena can be enlightening, they can also be unsettling for those unprepared for such encounters. Establishing a grounding practice, such as meditation or spending time in nature, helps individuals anchor their awareness amidst the vastness of psychic experiences, fostering a balanced and integrated approach.

Ego Dissolution: Kundalini's awakening often catalyzes a process of ego dissolution, challenging the individual's identification with the self. This dissolution of the ego can evoke a sense of existential crisis as individuals grapple with the impermanence of their self-concept. The fear of losing one's sense of identity can create resistance to the transformative process. Embracing practices that cultivate self-awareness, such as self-inquiry and mindfulness, allows individuals to navigate the dissolution of the ego with greater understanding and acceptance.

Lack of Guidance: Embarking on the Kundalini journey without adequate guidance can be a significant obstacle. The esoteric nature of Kundalini awakening requires a nuanced understanding of energy dynamics, spiritual principles, and the integration of higher states of consciousness. With proper guidance, individuals may feel safe and calm by the intensity of the experience. Seeking support from experienced mentors, teachers, or spiritual communities can provide invaluable insights and a sense of community, helping individuals navigate the intricacies of Kundalini activation with greater clarity and support.

Fear and Resistance: Fear stemming from the unknown or the intensity of Kundalini experiences can create resistance within the practitioner. The fear of losing control, facing the unknown, or encountering challenges may hinder the natural flow of Kundalini energy. Cultivating practices that address anxiety, such as mindfulness, breathwork, and affirmations, empower individuals to overcome resistance with courage and a deeper trust in the unfolding process.

In conclusion, while Kundalini awakening is a transformative journey leading to heightened awareness and self-realization, it is not exempt from challenges. Acknowledging and understanding these common obstacles allows individuals to approach their Kundalini journey with resilience, self-compassion, and a proactive mindset. Embracing the support of experienced mentors, integrating grounding practices, and fostering a holistic approach to well-being can contribute to a more harmonious and empowering experience of Kundalini activation. As practitioners navigate the complexities of this profound journey, the challenges encountered become opportunities for growth, self-discovery, and the unfolding of a deeper connection to the universal life force.

Strategies for overcoming challenges

Embarking on the transformative journey of Kundalini awakening is a profound and personal undertaking that may present various challenges. As individuals navigate the intricate pathways of heightened consciousness and energy ascension, developing strategies for overcoming the obstacles that may arise during this transformative process becomes essential. These strategies empower practitioners to navigate challenges with resilience, self-awareness, and purpose, fostering a harmonious and transformative Kundalini awakening experience.

Cultivating Mindfulness and Presence: A foundational strategy for overcoming challenges in Kundalini awakening is cultivating mindfulness and presence. By developing a heightened awareness of the present moment, practitioners can better navigate intense sensations, emotions, and psychic experiences. Conscious breathing and other mindfulness techniques, like meditation, provide skills for maintaining centering and grounding oneself in the face of energy and consciousness changes. Being mindful enables people to see the difficulties as they arise without becoming attached, which promotes stability and inner strength.

Grounding Practices: Grounding practices play a crucial role in overcoming challenges associated with the intensity of Kundalini energy. Anchoring the heightened energy in the physical body can be achieved by several techniques like going barefoot on natural surfaces, spending time in nature, or envisioning roots reaching into the earth. By offering steadiness and balance, grounding techniques help people avoid becoming overtaken by the energetic changes that come with Kundalini's awakening. Participating in grounding exercises regularly helps one experience the transformation process in a more integrated and centered way.

Establishing a Support System: Creating a support system is instrumental in overcoming challenges during Kundalini's awakening. Seeking guidance from experienced mentors, joining spiritual communities, or connecting with like-minded individuals who have undergone similar experiences fosters a sense of understanding and shared exploration. Having a support system provides a space for open dialogue, the exchange of insights, and mutual encouragement. This collaborative approach helps practitioners feel less isolated, reinforcing a sense of community and shared growth on the Kundalini path.

Integrating Holistic Practices: Integrating a variety of holistic practices supports the overall well-being of individuals undergoing Kundalini awakening. Complementary practices such as yoga, breathwork, sound healing, and bodywork contribute to a holistic approach, addressing the transformative journey's physical, emotional, and energetic aspects. Holistic practices create a synergistic effect, enhancing the overall resilience of the individual and providing diverse tools for navigating challenges. Integrating multiple modalities allows practitioners to tailor their approach to the unique dynamics of their Kundalini experience.

Seeking Professional Guidance: In some instances, seeking professional guidance from practitioners with expertise in Kundalini dynamics can offer valuable insights and support. Holistic healthcare professionals, energy healers, and spiritual mentors who understand the nuances of Kundalini awakening can provide guidance tailored to the individual's needs. This collaboration ensures that challenges are approached with a comprehensive understanding of the transformative process's energetic and physical aspects. Seeking professional guidance enhances practitioners' ability to navigate challenges with informed and personalized support.

Embracing a Fluid Approach: Adopting a fluid and adaptable approach is essential for overcoming challenges in Kundalini Awakening. The transformative journey is inherently dynamic, and experiences may vary from person to person. Embracing a fluid approach involves letting go of rigid expectations and allowing the process to unfold organically. This adaptability empowers practitioners to respond to challenges with creativity, resilience, and a willingness to explore new strategies as needed. By embracing the fluid nature of the Kundalini journey, individuals can navigate challenges with a sense of curiosity and openness.

Self-Reflection and Journaling: Engaging in regular self-reflection and journaling provides a valuable outlet for processing experiences, emotions, and insights encountered during Kundalini awakening. Writing allows individuals to explore their inner landscape, track patterns, and gain clarity on challenges that may arise. Journaling is a therapeutic tool for expressing thoughts and feelings, fostering a deeper understanding of the transformative journey. By cultivating self-awareness through reflective practices, practitioners can identify recurring challenges, track progress, and develop personalized strategies for overcoming obstacles.

Patience and Surrender: Cultivating patience and surrender is a fundamental strategy for overcoming challenges in Kundalini awakening. The transformative process unfolds at its own pace, and each individual's journey is unique. Practitioners are encouraged to embrace the ebb and flow of the Kundalini experience with patience, trusting in the innate wisdom of the process. Surrendering to the natural rhythm of the journey allows individuals to release resistance, reduce anxiety, and approach challenges with a sense of surrender to the transformative forces at play.

In conclusion, the strategies for overcoming challenges in Kundalini Awakening encompass a holistic and multifaceted approach. By integrating mindfulness, grounding practices, a support system, holistic modalities, professional guidance, adaptability, self-reflection, and patience, practitioners empower themselves to navigate the complexities of the transformative journey with resilience and grace. When these techniques are used, people have a complete arsenal to help them face obstacles with self-awareness, purpose, and an open heart, which promotes a peaceful and transformational Kundalini awakening experience.

Seeking guidance and support

Starting the transforming and complex process of Kundalini awakening frequently calls for help and direction. Activating dormant energy at the base of the spine is a sign of this spiritual journey, which can result in elevated states of consciousness and self-realization. Getting guidance becomes essential to guaranteeing a balanced and harmonious Kundalini awakening path as people traverse the intricacies of energetic shifts, expanded consciousness, and integrating spiritual experiences.

Mentorship and Experienced Guides: One of the primary avenues for seeking guidance in Kundalini Awakening is through mentorship and experienced guides. Those who have walked the path before, seasoned practitioners, or spiritual teachers with expertise in Kundalini dynamics can offer invaluable insights and support. The mentor-mentee relationship provides a personalized approach to understanding the nuances of the Kundalini journey. Experienced guides can guide navigating challenges, interpreting spiritual experiences, and maintaining balance during the transformative process. This mentorship fosters a sense of trust, allowing individuals to openly share their experiences and receive tailored advice based on the mentor's wisdom and firsthand knowledge.

Spiritual Communities and Support Groups: Engaging with spiritual communities and support groups dedicated to Kundalini awakening creates a sense of shared exploration and understanding. Online forums, local meet-ups, or gatherings organized by spiritual communities provide platforms for individuals to connect with like-minded seekers. Feelings of loneliness that might occasionally accompany the Kundalini journey are lessened by sharing experiences, insights, and difficulties with a caring group. These communities frequently include members at different phases of the awakening process, resulting in a rich tapestry of viewpoints and encouragement.

Professional Holistic Practitioners: Holistic practitioners with expertise in Kundalini dynamics, energy healing, and spiritual counseling offer experienced guidance for individuals undergoing Kundalini awakening. Energy healers, Reiki practitioners, and holistic counselors who understand the subtleties of energy work can provide personalized support. These practitioners may utilize modalities that align with the individual's needs, such as energy clearing, chakra balancing, and therapeutic counseling. Seeking guidance from holistic professionals ensures a comprehensive approach that considers both the energetic and emotional aspects of the Kundalini awakening journey.

Yoga and Meditation Instructors: Yoga and meditation instructors, mainly those well-versed in Kundalini Yoga, offer guidance on practices that enhance the Kundalini experience. With its specific postures, breathwork (pranayama), and meditations, Kundalini Yoga is designed to facilitate the safe and effective ascent of Kundalini energy. Instructors specializing in Kundalini Yoga can guide tailored practices to support the individual's unique journey. Regular attendance at Kundalini Yoga classes and workshops led by experienced instructors ensures a structured and supportive environment for practitioners to deepen their understanding and refine their practices.

Integration of Traditional Wisdom: Seeking guidance from sources rooted in traditional wisdom, such as ancient scriptures, texts, and teachings, offers a timeless and foundational approach to Kundalini awakening. Many spiritual traditions, including those within Hinduism, Buddhism, and Taoism, contain profound insights into the nature of consciousness, energy, and the spiritual path.

Individuals exploring Kundalini Awakening can benefit from studying these texts or seeking guidance from scholars and practitioners immersed in traditional wisdom. Integrating the timeless teachings from several traditions offers a more excellent knowledge of the spiritual path.

Therapeutic Support: Therapeutic support, including psychotherapy and counseling, can benefit individuals undergoing Kundalini awakening, especially when facing emotional or psychological challenges. Therapists trained in transpersonal psychology or who have an understanding of spiritual experiences can provide a safe space for individuals to explore the psychological aspects of their journey. Integrating therapeutic support alongside spiritual guidance ensures a holistic approach that addresses the Kundalini awakening process's spiritual and psychological dimensions.

Educational Resources and Workshops: Accessing educational resources and attending workshops on Kundalini Awakening contributes to an informed and empowered journey. Books, documentaries, online courses, and workshops led by reputable experts offer a wealth of information and practical guidance. These resources provide insights into the mechanics of Kundalini energy, the experiences associated with the awakening process, and strategies for navigating challenges. By continuously expanding their knowledge, individuals gain a deeper understanding of their experiences and can make informed decisions on their spiritual path.

Personal Reflection and Inner Guidance: While seeking external guidance is essential, cultivating personal reflection and inner guidance forms a foundational aspect of the Kundalini awakening journey. Meditation, introspection, and self-inquiry facilitate a direct connection with one's inner wisdom. Listening to the inner guidance that arises during stillness allows individuals to develop a profound understanding of their unique path. Trusting one's intuition and the innate intelligence of the Kundalini energy fosters a sense of self-empowerment and deepens the connection to the higher self.

In conclusion, seeking guidance and support is a dynamic and multifaceted aspect of the Kundalini awakening journey. The collaborative approach involving mentorship, spiritual communities, holistic practitioners, yoga instructors, traditional wisdom, therapeutic support, educational resources, and personal reflection creates a comprehensive support system for practitioners. Integrating external guidance with inner wisdom ensures a balanced, informed, and empowered approach to navigating the complexities of Kundalini awakening. As individuals open themselves to guidance from various sources, they create a rich tapestry of support that enhances their transformative journey toward self-realization and heightened consciousness.

CHAPTER VIII

Integrating Kundalini Energy into Daily Life

Balancing spiritual growth with everyday responsibilities

In the fast-paced and demanding landscape of modern life, individuals seeking spiritual growth often face the challenge of integrating their inner journey with the practical demands of everyday responsibilities. The quest for spiritual development, marked by introspection, mindfulness, and a deepening connection to the higher self, can sometimes seem at odds with the pressing obligations of work, family, and social commitments. However, the harmonious integration of spiritual practices into daily life enhances personal well-being and fosters a sense of purpose and fulfillment in navigating the world's complexities.

Navigating the delicate balance between spiritual growth and everyday responsibilities begins with a fundamental shift in perspective. Rather than viewing these two aspects of life as mutually exclusive, individuals can embrace the idea that spiritual practices can enrich and complement the fulfillment of daily duties. Recognizing the interconnected nature of the inner and outer realms creates a foundation for a holistic approach to living that integrates spiritual values into the fabric of daily existence.

Central to this integration is cultivating mindfulness in all aspects of life. Mindfulness, rooted in the present moment, allows individuals to bring a heightened awareness to their actions, thoughts, and interactions.

Whether engaged in professional tasks, familial responsibilities, or social interactions, mindfulness enables individuals to infuse each moment with a sense of presence and intention. By aligning everyday actions with spiritual principles such as compassion, gratitude, and authenticity, individuals can weave their spiritual growth seamlessly into the tapestry of their daily lives.

They are often perceived as mundane, practical routines that provide fertile ground for integrating spiritual practices. Consider the simple act of morning rituals—routines that set the tone for the day. Incorporating elements of mindfulness, such as conscious breathing, gratitude exercises, or short moments of reflection, transforms these rituals into opportunities for spiritual connection. By infusing intentionality into routine activities, individuals can create a sacred space within the ordinary, fostering a spiritual alignment throughout the day.

People spend many of their waking hours at work, so it presents a unique opportunity to balance personal and professional development. Integrating mindfulness into work tasks, adopting a compassionate approach to colleagues, and finding moments of stillness amidst busyness contribute to a spiritual presence in the workplace. Moreover, viewing work as an avenue for expressing one's values and contributing positively to the world elevates the mundane aspects of professional life to a higher purpose. The dichotomy between the spiritual and the practical dissolves when work becomes a form of mindful expression and service.

With its myriad responsibilities and relationships, family life presents challenges and opportunities for spiritual integration. It engages in conscious parenting, where moments of connection and presence precedence over distractions, and nurtures a spiritual connection within the family dynamic. Simple acts, such as sharing meals mindfully, expressing gratitude, and fostering open communication, become conduits for spiritual growth within the familial framework. Recognizing the inherent spiritual lessons embedded in domestic challenges encourages individuals to approach family life as a transformative journey.

Social interactions within communities or friendships offer further avenues for aligning spiritual growth with everyday engagements. Participating in conscious conversations, cultivating empathetic connections, and contributing positively to social circles become intentional acts of spiritual expression. By bringing authenticity, kindness, and compassion into social dynamics, individuals elevate their spiritual journey and contribute to their communities' collective well-being.

The art of balancing spiritual growth with everyday responsibilities also involves acknowledging the inevitability of challenges and setbacks. Life is inherently dynamic, and unforeseen circumstances may disrupt even well-established routines. During these challenging times, the integration of spiritual practices becomes a source of resilience and grounding. Individuals can navigate challenges with poise and adaptability by drawing upon the inner resources cultivated through mindfulness, introspection, and connection to a higher purpose.

Time management is a crucial component of striking a balance between daily obligations and spiritual development. It encourages people to give priority to pursuits that are consistent with their beliefs and enhance their well-being. Dedicating specific times for spiritual activities, such as prayer, meditation, or reflective writing, creates a regular pattern that fosters continued development.

Moreover, the cultivation of self-compassion plays a pivotal role in maintaining balance. Recognizing that spiritual growth is a gradual process and occasional deviations from routine are natural allows individuals to approach themselves with kindness rather than judgment. Self-compassion becomes a guiding force that encourages individuals to return to their spiritual practices with renewed dedication, fostering a sustainable and compassionate approach to integrating the spiritual and the practical.

In essence, balancing spiritual growth with everyday responsibilities is not about creating a rigid dichotomy but rather about weaving a seamless tapestry that encompasses both the sacred and the ordinary. Integrating spiritual practices into daily life is an ongoing journey that transforms routine activities into opportunities for mindfulness, compassion, and self-discovery. By approaching each moment with a heightened awareness and intentionality, individuals can navigate the complexities of the modern world while fostering a deep and meaningful connection to their spiritual essence. In this harmonious integration, pursuing spiritual growth becomes a transformative force that enriches every facet of life, creating a dynamic and purposeful existence.

Incorporating Kundalini practices into daily routines

The ancient wisdom of Kundalini, a potent form of spiritual energy believed to reside at the base of the spine, has captivated seekers on the path of self- realization for centuries. Kundalini practices, rooted in various Eastern spiritual traditions, offer a transformative journey of awakening and enlightenment. While the allure of this profound energy lies in its potential to unlock higher states of consciousness, integrating Kundalini practices into daily routines is a crucial aspect of harnessing and harmonizing this powerful force within the context of modern life.

The foundation of incorporating Kundalini practices into daily life begins with the recognition that spiritual growth is not confined to designated moments of meditation or ritualistic practices; instead, it is a dynamic and continuous process that can infuse every aspect of our existence. By investing Kundalini practices into daily routines, individuals create a sacred synergy between the inner and outer realms, fostering a harmonious and transformative way of living.

Morning Sadhana and Rituals: The morning serves as a potent canvas for setting the day's tone through the practice of Sadhana, a dedicated spiritual practice. Kundalini practitioners often engage in morning Sadhana, which typically includes a combination of Kundalini Yoga, meditation, mantra chanting, and breathwork. These practices are designed to awaken the dormant energy and align the practitioner with the higher self. Incorporating a personalized Sadhana into the morning routine creates a sacred space for communion with the divine, setting a positive and elevated tone for the day ahead.

Breathwork Throughout the Day: Conscious breathwork, or Pranayama, is a fundamental aspect of Kundalini practices. The breath bridges the physical and energetic dimensions, and incorporating conscious breathing into daily activities enhances awareness and vitality. Simple techniques, such as Breath of Fire or Long Deep Breathing, can be seamlessly woven into daily routines. Whether commuting, working at a desk, or engaging in household tasks, the conscious regulation of breath cultivates a sense of centeredness and presence, aligning the individual with the rhythmic flow of Kundalini energy.

Mindful Movement and Kundalini Yoga Breaks: Amid hectic schedules, incorporating short Kundalini Yoga breaks becomes a practical and rejuvenating way to infuse daily life with spiritual energy. With its unique postures, dynamic movements, and specific sequences, Kundalini Yoga is designed to awaken and channel the Kundalini energy. Integrating brief Kundalini Yoga sessions, even for a few minutes, offers an opportunity to release tension, enhance flexibility, and invigorate the energy centers. This mindful movement breaks contribute to overall well-being while providing a tangible experience of Kundalini's transformative potential.

Mantra and Chanting Practices: The vibrational power of mantra chanting is a potent tool for connecting with the spiritual dimensions of Kundalini energy. Incorporating mantra practices into daily routines, whether during a morning meditation or as a grounding ritual before bedtime, establishes a resonance with specific frequencies that elevate consciousness. Simple mantras, such as the universally powerful "Sat Nam" (Truth is my identity), can be recited silently or aloud, infusing daily activities with sacred vibrations and enhancing the practitioner's connection to the divine.

Mindful Eating and Nutrition: Eating is not only a physiological necessity but also an opportunity for mindful engagement with the energy of nourishment. Kundalini practitioners emphasize the importance of conscious eating, viewing food as a prana (life force energy) source. By approaching meals with gratitude, mindfulness, and an awareness of the energetic qualities of food, individuals can transform eating into a sacred act. This conscious approach to nutrition aligns the body's energy with the spiritual intent of Kundalini practices, promoting overall vitality and balance.

Evening Reflection and Meditation: As the day winds down, incorporating reflective practices and meditation creates a bridge between the outer activities and the inner realms. Evening meditation, whether guided or silent, allows individuals to process the day's experiences, release accumulated stress, and be attuned to the subtler currents of Kundalini energy. Creating a quiet and sacred space for evening reflection enhances the integration of

Kundalini practices into the daily rhythm, fostering a sense of completeness and inner harmony.

Intentional Transitions: Transitions between various activities provide opportunities to infuse mindfulness and Kundalini energy into daily routines. Whether transitioning from work to personal time, from one task to another, or wakefulness to sleep, consciously setting intentions and acknowledging the shifts in energy enhances the overall flow of Kundalini practices. Intentional transitions serve as reminders of the spiritual undercurrents that permeate daily life, encouraging a continuous awareness of the transformative journey.

Sacred Spaces and Altars: Creating a sacred space or altar within the living environment is a visual reminder of the spiritual commitment and connection to Kundalini practices. This designated space can be adorned with meaningful symbols, images, or objects that evoke a sense of reverence. Regularly spending time in this sacred space, whether for meditation, prayer, or quiet reflection, reinforces the integration of Kundalini practices into the daily routine, fostering a continuous and conscious connection to the divine.

Incorporating Kundalini practices into daily routines is a dynamic and creative process that transforms mundane activities into opportunities for spiritual awakening. By infusing everyday life with the vibrancy of Kundalini energy, individuals bridge the gap between the sacred and the ordinary, cultivating a holistic way of living that aligns with the transformative potential of this ancient wisdom. The harmonious integration of Kundalini practices into daily routines enhances individual well-being and fosters a deeper connection to the divine within the tapestry of modern life.

Nurturing ongoing spiritual development

The journey of spiritual development is a dynamic and continuous process, a pilgrimage of self-discovery that extends beyond momentary insights or fleeting revelations. Nurturing ongoing spiritual development involves cultivating a conscious and evolving relationship with the self, the divine, and the interconnected fabric of existence. Unlike a destination, spiritual growth is a perpetual voyage marked by deepening self-awareness, expanding consciousness, and an unwavering commitment to inner transformation. To embark on this profound journey and sustain it over time requires a multifaceted approach that integrates various practices, perspectives, and a deep understanding of the cyclical nature of growth.

At the heart of ongoing spiritual development lies the essence of self-awareness. This foundational quality serves as a compass, guiding individuals through the labyrinth of their inner landscapes. Cultivating self-awareness involves a continuous process of introspection, self-reflection, and a willingness to confront the layers of conditioning and egoic patterns that may obscure the true essence of one's being. Through meditation, mindfulness, and contemplation, individuals seek to understand the nature of their thoughts, emotions, and the subtle currents of consciousness that shape their experiences.

Understanding that spiritual growth occurs in cycles and stages, according to the seasons of nature, is essential to continuous spiritual progress. Accepting the cyclical nature of spiritual development enables people to handle life's ups and downs with acceptance and grace. There are times of expansion and revelation, where profound insights and spiritual breakthroughs occur, and there are times of contraction, where challenges and periods of inner gestation invite individuals to delve deeper into the recesses of their souls. The capacity to embrace both the light and shadow aspects of the journey fosters resilience, humility, and a holistic understanding of the transformative process.

A crucial aspect of nurturing ongoing spiritual development is the integration of spiritual practices into daily life. Consistent engagement in practices such as meditation, prayer, mindfulness, and energy work establish a rhythmic resonance with the spiritual dimensions. These practices serve as anchors, grounding individuals in the present moment while providing access to higher states of consciousness. By making these practices a part of daily routines, individuals create a sacred container for ongoing spiritual growth, fostering an environment where insights can blossom and the divine can be continually invited into their lives.

The concept of spiritual development extends beyond individual self-discovery to encompass the interconnectedness of all beings and the greater cosmos. Developing a sense of interconnectedness involves cultivating compassion, empathy, and a deep appreciation for the sacredness of all life. Kindness, service to others, and ecological awareness are integral components of ongoing spiritual development. Recognizing the interconnected web of existence, individuals understand that their spiritual journey is intricately woven with the collective journey of humanity and the planet's well-being.

Mindful engagement with life's challenges is another facet of nurturing ongoing spiritual development. Rather than viewing challenges as impediments to growth, individuals on the spiritual path approach them as opportunities for learning and transformation. Adversities become mirrors reflecting aspects of the self that require attention and healing. By embracing challenges with stability and a willingness to extract lessons from adversity, individuals catalyze profound shifts in consciousness, transcending limitations and deepening their spiritual understanding.

An essential companion to ongoing spiritual development is the cultivation of an open heart. Love, compassion, and forgiveness are expressions of the awakened heart and catalysts for spiritual growth. The practice of unconditional love extends not only to others but also to oneself. By releasing judgments, cultivating self-love, and developing compassion even in the face of personal challenges, individuals create a fertile ground for the seeds of spiritual development to flourish.

The mentorship and guidance of experienced spiritual teachers or wise mentors can play a pivotal role in nurturing ongoing spiritual development. These guides offer insights, wisdom, and practical advice based on their journeys. Their presence is a source of inspiration, providing clarity during moments of confusion and illumination during periods of darkness. Seeking the guidance of those who have traversed the spiritual path helps individuals navigate the nuances of their journey with a greater sense of purpose and direction.

Exploring diverse spiritual teachings and traditions contributes to the richness and diversity of ongoing spiritual development. While individuals may resonate with a particular tradition or philosophy, exploring various paths widens the spectrum of understanding and fosters a more inclusive and integrative approach to spirituality. One's spiritual viewpoint is expanded by interaction with sacred texts, spiritual meetings, and various practices; this enables a more thorough and nuanced understanding of the spiritual path.

The practice of gratitude is a transformative force in nurturing ongoing spiritual development. Cultivating gratitude involves recognizing and appreciating every moment's blessings, lessons, and gifts. Gratitude acts as a magnetic force, drawing more positive and transformative experiences into one's life. By acknowledging the interconnectedness of all experiences and expressing gratitude for both challenges and blessings, individuals create a harmonious resonance that propels them forward on their spiritual journey.

In conclusion, nurturing ongoing spiritual development is a profound and dynamic commitment to self-discovery, growth, and realizing one's divine potential. It involves a holistic approach that integrates self-awareness, the cyclical nature of growth, daily spiritual practices, interconnectedness, mindful engagement with challenges, an open heart, guidance from mentors, exploration of diverse teachings, and the transformative power of gratitude. By embracing the multifaceted nature of the spiritual journey, individuals deepen their understanding of themselves and contribute to the collective evolution of consciousness, fostering a more awakened and compassionate world.

CHAPTER IX

The Spiritual Evolution

The profound impact of Kundalini awakening on spiritual evolution

Kundalini awakening, a phenomenon deeply rooted in Eastern spiritual traditions, represents a pinnacle in the journey of spiritual evolution. This extraordinary experience is often described as the activation of dormant, coiled energy at the base of the spine, surging upward through the chakras and unlocking higher states of consciousness. The impact of Kundalini's awakening on spiritual evolution is profound, ushering individuals into a realm of expanded awareness, heightened perception, and direct communion with the divine.

At its core, Kundalini awakening is a catalyst for the evolution of consciousness—a transformative force that propels individuals beyond the boundaries of ordinary perception. The awakening of the dormant Kundalini energy initiates a process of purification and illumination, clearing energetic blockages and aligning the subtle body with the flow of divine energy. As this potent energy ascends through the chakra system, it activates and harmonizes the various energy centers, profoundly restructuring the individual's inner landscape.

One of the hallmark effects of Kundalini's awakening is the amplification of spiritual experiences and insights. The heightened sensitivity of the awakened nervous system allows individuals to perceive subtle energies, access higher realms of consciousness, and experience a deep sense of interconnectedness with all of creation. Spiritual revelations, once veiled, become more accessible, leading to a profound understanding of the underlying unity and oneness that permeates the fabric of existence.

The impact of Kundalini's awakening extends beyond personal experience, influencing how individuals engage with the world around them. The heightened awareness and expanded consciousness foster a sense of reverence for all of life. Individuals undergoing Kundalini awakening often develop a deep appreciation for the interconnected web of existence, recognizing the divine essence within every being and every manifestation of creation. This shift in perception lays the foundation for a more compassionate, mindful, and ecologically conscious way of living.

The transformative effects of Kundalini's awakening on spiritual evolution also manifest in the dissolution of egoic structures and the liberation from conditioned patterns of thought and behavior. The surge of Kundalini's energy dismantles the constructs of the ego, leading to a profound shift in identity and a reorientation toward the higher self. As individuals become attuned to the purifying force of Kundalini, they often experience a deep sense of ego dissolution. This ego death paves a rebirth into a more authentic and spiritually aligned expression of self. Kundalini awakening acts as a potent catalyst for inner alchemy, transmuting the lead of human consciousness into the gold of spiritual illumination. The energy released during the awakening process purifies and rejuvenates the entire system, enhancing physical, mental, and emotional well-being. Individuals often report increased vitality, heightened creativity, and a sense of inner peace that transcends the fluctuations of external circumstances. The transformative impact on the physical and energetic bodies is a testament to the potency of Kundalini energy and an affirmation of the inseparable connection between mind, body, and spirit.

The awakening of Kundalini also catalyzes the activation of latent spiritual potentials, unlocking abilities and gifts that lie dormant within the individual. Heightened intuition, extrasensory perceptions, and a deepened connection to higher guidance become more accessible to those undergoing Kundalini awakening. This expansion of spiritual capacities is not meant to be wielded as mere personal accomplishments but as tools for service, aiding individuals in contributing to the greater good and the collective evolution of consciousness.

A significant aspect of the impact of Kundalini's awakening on spiritual evolution is the deepening connection to the divine source. The awakened Kundalini serves as a conduit for the direct experience of the divine within. Individuals undergoing this transformative process often describe profound communion with the divine, experiencing a sense of oneness and unity that transcends religious or cultural boundaries. The direct, unmediated connection to the sacred becomes a guiding force in the individual's spiritual evolution, fostering a deepening relationship with the divine's transcendent and immanent aspects.

It is essential to acknowledge that the journey of Kundalini awakening has challenges. Kundalini's purifying and transformative energies can stir the depths of the unconscious, bringing to the surface unresolved emotions, traumas, and shadow aspects of the self. This process of purification, though challenging, is an integral part of the spiritual evolution facilitated by Kundalini awakening. It invites individuals to confront and release the layers of conditioning that obstruct the free flow of divine energy, leading to a more authentic and liberated expression of self.

In conclusion, the profound impact of Kundalini's awakening on spiritual evolution is a testament to the transformative power of this ancient spiritual phenomenon. The awakening of the dormant Kundalini energy initiates a journey of heightened awareness, expanded consciousness, and direct communion with the divine. The ripple effects of Kundalini awakening extend into all dimensions of life, influencing perception, identity, well-being, and how individuals engage with the world. As a catalyst for inner alchemy, the awakening of Kundalini unlocks latent potentials and gifts, propelling individuals toward a more authentic and spiritually aligned expression of self. Embracing both the challenges and blessings of this transformative process, individuals on the path of Kundalini awakening contribute to their own evolution and the collective awakening of human consciousness.

Connecting with higher consciousness

The quest for higher consciousness is an ageless journey transcending cultural, religious, and philosophical boundaries. Rooted in the inherent human yearning for transcendence and a deeper understanding of existence, pursuing higher consciousness involves reaching beyond the confines of ordinary perception to access a profound, elevated state of awareness. This journey is not merely a personal endeavor but a universal exploration that seeks to unveil the mysteries of the cosmos, the nature of the self, and the interconnectedness of all things. Connecting with higher consciousness is a transformative process that invites individuals to transcend the limitations of the ego, expand their perception, and attune to the vibrational frequencies of the divine.

At the heart of connecting with higher consciousness lies the recognition that the human experience extends beyond the physical and material realms. The ancient wisdom traditions have long asserted that the true nature of selfhood is not confined to the transient physical body but is an expression of a timeless, formless essence. In pursuing higher consciousness, individuals embark on an inner journey to explore and experience this essential aspect of self—the divine spark that animates all creation. This recognition catalyzes a shift in perception, inviting individuals to see beyond the illusion of separateness and embrace the interconnected oneness that underlies the tapestry of existence.

Meditation, a practice in various spiritual traditions, is a potent gateway to connecting with higher consciousness. Through meditation, individuals enter into a state of focused awareness, quieting the constant chatter of the mind and creating space for a direct experience of the transcendent. Whether through mindfulness meditation, loving-kindness meditation, or contemplative practices, individuals cultivate a receptive state of consciousness that allows them to connect with the deeper layers of their being and tap into the universal field of higher awareness.

Contemplating the profound mysteries of existence is another avenue for connecting with higher consciousness. This intellectual and spiritual inquiry involves delving into questions that surpass the boundaries of conventional understanding and exploring the nature of reality, the purpose of life, and the dynamics of the cosmos. The pursuit of wisdom through contemplation serves as a bridge between the rational mind and intuitive knowing, leading individuals to insights that transcend the limitations of ordinary cognition and open doors to higher realms of understanding.

Exploring altered states of consciousness, whether induced through meditation, breathwork, or other contemplative practices, provides a unique opportunity to connect with higher dimensions of awareness. These altered states, often characterized by expanded perception, enhanced intuition, and a sense of timelessness, allow individuals to experience the interconnected web of existence more directly and viscerally. The dissolution of the boundaries between self and other, subject and object, creates a profound sense of unity with the cosmos, fostering a connection with higher consciousness that transcends the limitations of the egoic mind.

Sacred rituals and ceremonies, deeply ingrained in various cultural and spiritual traditions, offer a ceremonial space for connecting with higher consciousness. Whether through prayer, chanting, or symbolic gestures, these rituals serve as portals facilitating a sacred communion with the divine. The repetition of holy words, the rhythm of ritualistic movements, and the intentional creation of sacred space create a vibrational resonance that elevates individual and collective consciousness, fostering a sense of unity with the transcendent.

With its intricate beauty and profound interconnectedness, the natural world is a powerful catalyst for connecting with higher consciousness. Immersing oneself in nature through contemplative walks, ecological mindfulness, or simply communing with the elements allows individuals to attune to the inherent wisdom and harmonious energy that permeate the natural world. The interconnected web of life becomes a mirror reflecting the more profound unity that transcends the diversity of forms, providing a tangible and immediate experience of higher consciousness.

Engaging in practices cultivating compassion and unconditional love is a transformative pathway to connecting with higher consciousness. The vibrational frequency of love, described as the highest and most refined state of consciousness in various spiritual traditions, opens the heart and aligns individuals with the divine essence. Acts of kindness, selfless service, and the intentional cultivation of a loving presence create a resonance with higher realms of consciousness, inviting individuals to embody the qualities of the divine in their daily lives.

The wisdom of the ages, preserved in sacred texts, scriptures, and teachings, offers a profound resource for connecting with higher consciousness. Delving into the timeless wisdom found in traditions such as Advaita Vedanta, Sufism, Kabbalah, and mystical Christianity provides individuals with insights and guidance that transcend the limitations of temporal knowledge. These teachings serve as a roadmap for the inner journey, offering principles and practices that facilitate the direct experience of higher states of consciousness.

Dreamwork and the exploration of the subconscious realms also play a role in connecting with higher consciousness. Dreams, often considered a bridge between the conscious and unconscious mind, offer a symbolic language through which higher guidance and insights can be conveyed. The practice of lucid dreaming or intentional dream exploration becomes a means for individuals to access the deeper layers of the psyche and receive messages from the higher self or spiritual guides. In essence, connecting with higher consciousness is a multi-faceted and transformative journey that integrates meditation, contemplation, altered states of consciousness, sacred rituals, communion with nature, acts of love and compassion, wisdom from holy texts, and the exploration of dreams. This holistic approach recognizes that higher consciousness is not a distant goal to be reached but a timeless dimension that can be accessed through various portals within the human experience. As individuals embark on this profound journey, they discover that connecting with higher consciousness is a personal endeavor and a universal quest that aligns them with the eternal dance of cosmic evolution, guiding them toward a more awakened and enlightened way of being.

Embracing the journey of continuous growth

The journey of continuous growth is a sacred pilgrimage that weaves its threads through the tapestry of human existence. It is an odyssey that transcends the boundaries of time, a perpetual unfolding that beckons individuals to navigate the ever-shifting landscapes of self-discovery, learning, and evolution. At its essence, embracing the journey of continuous growth is a commitment to the dynamic process of becoming, acknowledging that self-discovery is not a destination but a sacred unfolding that invites us to dance with the rhythm of life's perpetual changes.

Central to embracing continuous growth is recognizing that growth is not confined to specific phases of life but is an inherent and lifelong process. From birth until the final breath, the human experience is marked by an unfolding tapestry of experiences, challenges, and learning opportunities. Embracing continuous growth requires a shift in perspective, a willingness to see every moment as a potential catalyst for expansion, and a recognition that the journey of growth is not linear but spirals through the cycles of renewal and transformation.

The foundation of the journey of continuous growth lies in cultivating a growth mindset—a mental framework that views challenges as opportunities, failures as stepping stones, and the unknown as a fertile ground for exploration. Individuals with a growth mindset approach life with curiosity, resilience, and a willingness to stretch beyond their comfort zones. This mindset fosters a sense of agency, as individuals recognize that their efforts, attitudes, and commitment to learning contribute to their personal and collective growth.

Education, in its broadest sense, becomes a vital ally in continuous growth. Beyond formal schooling, pursuing knowledge and wisdom becomes a lifelong endeavor. Whether through books, mentors, experiences, or self-directed learning, individuals on the path of continuous growth pursue a perpetual quest for understanding, insight, and the refinement of their intellectual and emotional capacities. The hunger for knowledge becomes a guiding force, propelling individuals toward deeper realms of experience and a more profound engagement with the mysteries of existence.

The journey of continuous growth is intrinsically connected to self-awareness—a dynamic and ongoing process of exploring the depths of one's psyche, motivations, and behavior patterns. Through meditation, introspection, and mindfulness, individuals cultivate a heightened awareness of their thoughts, emotions, and the subtle currents of consciousness that shape their experiences. This self-awareness becomes a compass, guiding individuals through the labyrinth of their inner landscapes and unveiling the layers of conditioning that may obstruct their growth path.

Challenges and obstacles are not viewed as hindrances on the journey of continuous growth but as stepping stones that catalyze transformation. The transformative power of adversity lies in its ability to unearth latent potentials, resilience, and hidden strengths within individuals. Embracing challenges as opportunities for growth reframes setbacks as invitations to evolve, learn, and emerge stronger on the other side. This mindset shift empowers individuals to navigate the complexities of life with grace and poise.

Relationships with oneself and others play a pivotal role in the journey of continuous growth. Interactions with diverse individuals become mirrors reflecting aspects of the self that may require attention, healing, or integration. Healthy relationships become crucibles for personal and relational growth, inviting individuals to develop empathy, compassion, and effective communication. The tapestry of human connection becomes a fertile ground for learning as individuals navigate intimacy, collaboration, and mutual understanding.

The journey of continuous growth is not solely an individual pursuit but is woven into the collective fabric of humanity. Recognizing our interconnectedness with others and the world at large fosters a sense of responsibility for the well-being of the joint. Social and ecological consciousness become integral to the journey, prompting individuals to contribute to the greater good and co-create a more just, compassionate, and sustainable world.

Spirituality becomes a guiding light in continuous growth, providing individuals with a deeper context for their experiences and a connection to something greater than themselves. Whether through religious practices, mystical traditions, or a personal relationship with the divine, spirituality infuses the journey with meaning, purpose, and a sense of the sacred. The quest for spiritual growth becomes a transformative current that guides individuals toward realizing their highest potential and a more profound understanding of the nature of existence. Embracing the journey of continuous growth necessitates a certain degree of surrender—an openness to the unknown and a willingness to release attachments to fixed outcomes. The journey's fluidity necessitates that people flow with life's constantly shifting currents, learning from and maturing in reaction to the ups and downs of events. This surrender is not a passive resignation but an active participation in the dance of life, a recognition that growth often unfolds in unexpected ways and through unanticipated avenues.

In conclusion, embracing the journey of continuous growth is a profound invitation to dance with life's rhythms, navigate the ever-shifting landscapes of self- discovery, and engage in the perpetual process of becoming. It is a commitment to a growth mindset, a dedication to lifelong learning, and a recognition that challenges, relationships, and spirituality are integral aspects of the journey. The journey of continuous growth is not a linear path but a spiraling odyssey that invites individuals to stretch beyond their comfort zones, cultivate self-awareness, navigate challenges with resilience, and contribute to the collective evolution of humanity. In embracing continuous growth, individuals discover that the journey is the destination. This sacred pilgrimage unfolds with every breath, inviting them to blossom into the fullest expression of their human potential.

CHAPTER X

Stories of Transformation

Real-life accounts of individuals who experienced Kundalini awakening

Kundalini awakening, a transformative and often mysterious process rooted in ancient spiritual traditions, has captured the attention and curiosity of seekers throughout the ages. While the concept of Kundalini is deeply ingrained in the esoteric traditions of Yoga, Tantra, and various Eastern philosophies, its manifestation is not confined to the pages of sacred texts. Real-life accounts of individuals who have undergone Kundalini awakening offer a glimpse into the profound and sometimes challenging nature of this extraordinary spiritual experience.

One common thread in these accounts is Kundalini's awakening's spontaneous and unexpected nature. Many individuals report that the awakening process was not initiated through deliberate spiritual practices but unfolded spontaneously, often catching them by surprise. It might be triggered by intense meditation, moments of deep contemplation, or even life-altering events. The unpredictability of Kundalini's awakening underscores its organic and non-linear nature, challenging preconceived notions about the deliberate control one might have over such a potent spiritual force.

For those who have experienced Kundalini awakening, the opening of the energetic pathways is often accompanied by intense physical sensations. Heat, vibrations, and a surge of energy moving through the spine are commonly reported. Some people say having the sensation of a strong force ascending from the base of their spine to the top of their head. These bodily sensations are not merely physical but are intertwined with a profound sense of inner alchemy, as if the body's very cells are undergoing a purification and realignment process.

Emotional and psychological shifts are prevalent aspects of Kundalini awakening, as reported by those who have undergone this experience. The release of stored emotions, unresolved traumas, and deep-seated fears can surface, demanding conscious attention and integration. Individuals often describe a rollercoaster of emotions ranging from ecstatic bliss to moments of profound darkness. The psychological landscape becomes a terrain for exploration, inviting individuals to confront and transcend the layers of conditioning that may obstruct the free flow of Kundalini energy.

The opening of the psychic faculties is another dimension frequently encountered in real-life accounts of Kundalini's awakening. Heightened intuition, extrasensory perceptions, and a deepened connection to the subtle realms of existence become more accessible. Some individuals report clairvoyant visions, telepathic experiences, or a heightened sensitivity to the energies of others. Expanding psychic capacities is not seen as an end but a means for individuals to navigate the spiritual dimensions with greater clarity and insight.

The impact of Kundalini's awakening on one's worldview is often profound. Individuals describe a fundamental shift in their perception of reality, transcending the limitations of dualistic thinking. One experiences the unity and connection that underlie all creation as the barriers between self and other, subject and object, vanish. The mundane aspects of life take on a heightened significance, and individuals often report a deepened reverence for the sacredness inherent in every moment.

However, the journey of Kundalini awakening has its challenges. Real-life accounts reveal that the intensified energy flow can be overwhelming, leading to physical discomfort, sleep disturbances, and disruptions in daily life. Unearthing suppressed emotions and unresolved issues can also bring individuals face-to-face with their shadow aspects, necessitating a process of conscious integration. The delicate balance between the expansive and contractive forces within the awakening process requires individuals to navigate the path with discernment and self-care.

Spiritual crises, known as Kundalini crises, are reported by some individuals undergoing awakening. These crises can manifest as intense physical and emotional upheaval periods, sometimes leading individuals to question their sanity or face existential doubts. While challenging, these crises are viewed in some spiritual traditions as necessary purifications, burning away the egoic self's dross to reveal the true self's luminosity beneath.

Despite the challenges, real-life accounts of Kundalini's awakening often highlight the profound positive transformations that individuals undergo. Many report a deepening connection to their spiritual essence, an expanded capacity for love and compassion, and a sense of purpose that transcends the egoic desires of the lower self. Integrating the awakened Kundalini energy aligns individuals with their higher selves, guiding them toward self-realization and spiritual evolution.

One recurrent theme in these accounts is the importance of guidance and support during the Kundalini awakening process. Seekers often turn to spiritual mentors, experienced practitioners, or communities of like-minded individuals to navigate the complexities of the journey. Sharing experiences with others who have undergone

Kundalini awakening fosters a sense of validation, understanding, and the reassurance that one is not alone in the challenges and blessings of the awakening process.

In conclusion, real-life accounts of individuals who have experienced Kundalini awakening paint a nuanced picture of this extraordinary spiritual phenomenon. The spontaneous and unpredictable nature of the awakening, coupled with intense physical, emotional, and psychic shifts, underscores the potency and transformative power of Kundalini energy. The journey is not without its challenges, yet the positive transformations, deepened spiritual connection and profound shifts in perception reveal the potential for profound self-realization and spiritual evolution. As these real-life stories illuminate, Kundalini's awakening is a multi-faceted journey that invites individuals to dance with the sacred fire within, embracing the complexities and mysteries of their spiritual unfoldment.

Lessons learned, and insights gained

Life's journey is a profound school, a continuous unfolding of experiences that shape, mold, and, ultimately, offer profound lessons for those willing to embrace them. Every meeting, difficulty, and victory people encounter during their odysseys serve as stepping stones toward developing a more profound sense of self-awareness and wisdom. Reflecting on the lessons learned and insights gained throughout life's journey illuminates the transformative power embedded in every experience, offering a roadmap for personal growth, resilience, and the cultivation of a deeper understanding of the human condition.

One fundamental lesson that life consistently imparts is the inevitability of change. The impermanence of all things is a poignant reminder that, like the ebb and flow of tides, life is in constant flux. Embracing change as a natural and essential aspect of existence allows individuals to navigate uncertainties with extraordinary grace and adaptability. The ability to flow with the river of life rather than resisting its currents becomes a profound skill, opening doors to new opportunities, perspectives, and the continual self-renewal process.

Often viewed as an unwelcome intruder, adversity is revealed through reflection as a wise and compassionate teacher. Each challenge, setback, or moment of discomfort holds the potential for growth and transformation within it. The insights gained through adversity are not merely intellectual but engraved in the fabric of one's being, fostering resilience, courage, and the unwavering capacity to rise anew after each fall. As the Japanese proverb wisely states, "Fall seven times, stand up eight."

Self-awareness emerges as a cornerstone lesson in the journey of life. Exploring one's inner landscape, motivations, fears, and aspirations becomes a sacred pilgrimage. Through introspection, individuals uncover the layers of conditioning, societal expectations, and limiting beliefs that shape their perceptions of self and the world. This self-discovery continually unfolds, inviting individuals to peel away the layers and reveal the authentic core beneath.

The interplay between connection and solitude becomes a vital lesson in the intricate dance of human relationships. While connection nourishes the soul and provides a mirror for self-discovery, solitude serves as a crucible for introspection, creativity, and the cultivation of inner strength. Balancing these dual aspects of the human experience allows individuals to engage authentically with others while maintaining a grounded connection to their essence.

One of life's most important lessons through the fabric of relationships is empathy—the capacity to comprehend and experience another person's feelings. Walking in another's shoes fosters compassion and nurtures the seeds of a more harmonious world. Recognizing that everyone carries their own burdens, joys, and unique journey of self-discovery cultivates a spirit of understanding and unity, transcending the illusion of separateness.

Time, a finite and precious resource, imparts the lesson of mindful presence. The recognition that the present moment is all that truly exists encourages individuals to savor the richness of each experience rather than dwelling on the past or anxiously anticipating the future. Mindful presence becomes a gateway to a deeper engagement with life, fostering gratitude, joy, and a profound sense of aliveness.

The pursuit of knowledge and the embrace of curiosity emerge as invaluable companions on the journey of life. Recognizing that every encounter, whether joyful or challenging, holds the potential for learning within it fosters a growth mindset. The willingness to explore the mysteries of existence, question assumptions, and seek understanding becomes a guiding force, propelling individuals toward intellectual and spiritual evolution.

Forgiveness, a profound act of self-liberation, stands as a transformative lesson in the human journey. The ability to release resentment, judgment, and the weight of past grievances allows individuals to reclaim their emotional freedom. Forgiveness is not an endorsement of wrongdoing but a recognition that holding onto anger and resentment only perpetuates one's suffering. Through forgiveness, individuals pave the way for healing, liberation, and possibly creating a more compassionate world.

Love, the most potent force in the universe, reveals itself as life's ultimate lesson and purpose. Cultivation and expression of love for oneself and others are accurate measures of a well-lived life. Love transcends the boundaries of time and space, nurturing the seeds of connection, compassion, and a profound sense of interconnectedness with all creation.

In conclusion, the lessons learned and insights gained through the journey of life are as diverse and nuanced as the myriad experiences that shape an individual's existence. Embracing change, finding wisdom in adversity, cultivating self-awareness, balancing connection and solitude, practicing empathy, valuing time, nurturing curiosity, embracing forgiveness, and ultimately, embodying love are among the profound lessons that life imparts. As individuals reflect on these lessons, they uncover a roadmap for personal growth, resilience, and the cultivation of a meaningful and purposeful existence. Life's journey is a continual invitation to dance with the wisdom embedded in every moment, learn from the rich tapestry of experiences, and embody the profound lessons illuminating the path toward a more conscious and fulfilling life.

Inspiration for those on their own Kundalini journey

Embarking on the path of Kundalini awakening is akin to stepping into the heart of a transformative and mysterious journey that unfolds within the realms of the physical, emotional, and spiritual dimensions. For those treading the path of the awakened serpent energy, the Kundalini journey is both a sacred pilgrimage and an exploration of the boundless potential of human consciousness. As seekers navigate the ebbs and flows of this profound process, drawing inspiration becomes an essential companion, offering guidance, solace, and encouragement. Through recognizing the difficulties, appreciating the gifts, and highlighting the transformative potential inherent in this holy quest, this section seeks to offer guidance and encouragement to those on their own Kundalini trip.

First and foremost, it is crucial to recognize the uniqueness of each Kundalini journey. No two paths are identical, for the serpent energy weaves its way through the intricate tapestry of an individual's life, touching upon the specific nuances of their experiences, challenges, and revelations. Embracing the uniqueness of one's journey fosters a sense of acceptance and allows seekers to honor their own rhythm and pace in the unfolding process of Kundalini's awakening.

A foundational inspiration for those on the Kundalini journey lies in the understanding that the awakening of this potent energy is a natural and inherent aspect of human evolution. Drawing on ancient spiritual traditions and sacred texts, the image of Kundalini energy is often that of a sleeping serpent curled up at the base of the spine, ready to be aroused. Recognizing the innate potential for spiritual awakening within each individual is an empowering realization. It shifts the perspective from perceiving Kundalini's awakening as an esoteric or unattainable experience to understanding it as a birthright—an integral part of the human journey toward self-realization.

The rich tapestry of ancient wisdom, encompassing various traditions such as Yoga, Tantra, and Eastern mysticism, serves as a wellspring of inspiration for those traversing the Kundalini path. These traditions provide maps, practices, and guidance accumulated over centuries, offering seekers a framework to understand and navigate the intricacies of the awakening process. Delving into these timeless teachings provides valuable insights and connects individuals to a lineage of wisdom keepers who have trod the same path throughout history. The interconnectedness of the Kundalini journey with the broader human experience becomes another source of inspiration. Recognizing that the challenges and joys encountered on this path echo the universal themes of growth, transformation, and self-discovery fosters a sense of kinship with humanity. In the shared journey of awakening, individuals find solace, realizing that they are not alone in their experiences. This recognition of shared humanity creates a sense of community and support within and beyond those actively engaged in Kundalini awakening.

Another profound inspiration on the Kundalini journey is the transformative power embedded in the challenges encountered. The awakening of Kundalini's energy is not a linear progression but often involves unearthing suppressed emotions, unresolved traumas, and deep-seated fears. While these challenges may seem daunting, they are viewed in spiritual traditions as opportunities for purification and growth. Embracing the difficulties as catalysts for inner transformation allows seekers to navigate the journey with resilience, courage, and a deepened understanding of the self.

The experiences of real-life individuals who have undergone Kundalini awakening offer invaluable inspiration for those on the path. Stories of spontaneous awakenings, personal triumphs, and the integration of Kundalini energy into daily life serve as beacons of light, illuminating the possibilities and potentials of the journey. These narratives provide insights into the multifaceted nature of Kundalini's awakening, acknowledging its ecstatic moments and possible challenges. Exploring these accounts fosters a sense of hope, guidance, and reassurance for those traversing their unique paths.

The symbiotic relationship between Kundalini awakening and spiritual practices becomes a wellspring of inspiration. While awakening is often spontaneous, various contemplative practices, breathwork, meditation, and yogic disciplines are recognized as supportive tools. Engaging in these practices with sincerity and devotion becomes a way to cultivate receptivity to the awakening energy and create a conducive inner environment. Integrating spiritual practices into daily life serves as a reminder that the Kundalini journey is not solely about reaching a destination but involves a continual process of refinement, alignment, and atonement.

Seekers on the Kundalini journey draw inspiration from the deepened connection to higher states of consciousness and expanded awareness that often accompanies the awakening process. The opening of the energetic pathways and the activation of subtle faculties allow individuals to glimpse the interconnectedness of all existence. This expanded awareness fosters a reverence for the sacredness inherent in every moment and a recognition of the divine presence within and around them. The inspiration derived from these transcendent experiences propels seekers toward a more profound understanding of the nature of reality.

Acknowledging the transformative potential of Kundalini awakening in the context of healing and self-discovery becomes another source of inspiration. As the serpent energy moves through the chakras, it is believed to purify and harmonize the energetic centers, bringing about a profound healing of the physical, emotional, and spiritual dimensions. Individuals often report a sense of wholeness, balance, and newfound clarity in navigating their inner landscapes. The inspiration derived from the healing aspects of Kundalini awakening encourages seekers to view the journey as a holistic process that integrates the fragmented elements of the self.

The understanding that Kundalini's awakening is not confined to a specific timeframe but unfolds by one's readiness becomes a source of patience and inspiration. The serpent energy respects the natural rhythm of an individual's evolution, and the timing of the awakening is often influenced by various factors, including one's spiritual maturity, life circumstances, and past karmic imprints. Embracing patience becomes an essential aspect of the Kundalini journey, allowing seekers to surrender to the divine timing of the awakening process.

In conclusion, the Kundalini journey is a sacred and transformative odyssey that invites individuals to dance with the serpentine energy within. Drawing inspiration from the uniqueness of one's path, the rich tapestry of ancient wisdom, the interconnectedness with humanity, the transformative power of challenges, real-life accounts, spiritual practices, expanded awareness, healing potential, and the patient surrender to the unfolding process illuminates the path for those on their own Kundalini journey. As seekers navigate the twists and turns of this profound odyssey, may they find solace, guidance, and a deepened connection to the infinite possibilities that await within the awakened serpent energy. The Kundalini journey is not just a personal exploration but an invitation to participate in the cosmic dance of awakening, contributing to the collective evolution of human consciousness.

CHAPTER XI

Beyond Kundalini Awakening

Exploring advanced spiritual practices

As individuals traverse the expansive landscapes of their spiritual journey, a profound yearning often arises to explore advanced spiritual practices. These practices go beyond the introductory stages of meditation and essential mindfulness, delving into esoteric knowledge, mystical experiences, and a deeper communion with the divine. Advanced spiritual practices are not meant for everyone, as they require a foundation of spiritual maturity, self-discipline, and a genuine commitment to self-realization. This section explores various advanced spiritual practices, their significance, and the potential transformative power they hold for those who embark on the sacred journey of exploration.

One of the central pillars of advanced spiritual practices is the exploration of altered states of consciousness. While meditation lays the groundwork for heightened awareness, advanced practitioners often seek to transcend ordinary states of perception and access altered realms of reality. Techniques such as deep trance meditation, lucid dreaming, or entheogenic substances are avenues through which seekers may temporarily shift their consciousness, gaining access to insights, visions, and experiences beyond ordinary sensory perception. The careful and responsible exploration of altered states can catalyze expanded awareness and a deeper understanding of the nature of reality.

Tantric practices, rooted in ancient Eastern traditions, represent another facet of advanced spiritual exploration. Tantra, often associated with sacred sexuality, encompasses a broader spectrum of practices that seek to harness and transmute the powerful energies within the human system. Advanced tantric rituals involve the awakening and circulation of Kundalini energy, channeling sexual energy for spiritual transformation, and the integration of polarities within the self. These practices are not for the faint of heart, requiring a deep understanding of the energetic anatomy, a harmonious relationship with one's sexuality, and guidance from experienced mentors.

Pursuing direct mystical experiences is a hallmark of advanced spiritual practices. While many spiritual traditions offer maps and practices to cultivate heightened awareness, advanced seekers often yearn for a direct and unmediated encounter with the divine. Practices such as contemplative prayer, deep meditation, or Sufi whirling may serve as gateways to mystical states where the boundaries between the self and the divine blur. The mystic seeks knowledge about the holy and a direct, experiential communion that transcends intellectual understanding.

Often shrouded in mystery and symbolism, Esoteric traditions beckon advanced seekers into the depths of hidden knowledge. Alchemy, Qabalah, and Hermeticism are examples of esoteric systems that delve into spirituality's arcane and mystical aspects. These practices involve the study of ancient texts, symbolic interpretations, and the application of transformative rituals. Exploring esoteric knowledge requires a discerning mind and a willingness to unravel the hidden meanings encoded in ancient wisdom, inviting seekers to become alchemists of their spiritual evolution.

Culturing psychic abilities becomes a natural progression for those engaged in advanced spiritual practices. Clairvoyance, telepathy, and psychometry are among the various psychic faculties that advanced practitioners may seek to develop. These abilities are viewed not as ends but as tools for navigating the subtle dimensions of existence and gaining deeper insights into the interconnected nature of reality. The responsible development of psychic abilities requires humility, ethical considerations, and a commitment to serving the greater good.

Sadhana, or spiritual discipline, is intensified in advanced spiritual practices. The commitment to a daily practice becomes a means of self-purification and a conscious engagement with the divine. Advanced seekers may incorporate rigorous disciplines such as extended periods of silent retreat, intensive mantra chanting, or prolonged periods of fasting into their sadhana. These practices purify the mind, body, and spirit, creating a vessel receptive to the higher frequencies of spiritual realization.

Exploring sacred geometry and its application in spiritual practices forms another dimension of advanced exploration. Sacred geometry, with its intricate patterns and mathematical precision, is believed to be a key to understanding the underlying order of the cosmos. Practices involving mandalas, yantras, or labyrinth walking are ways in which seekers engage with the geometric language of the universe, tapping into the harmonizing principles that govern creation.

The study and application of sound as a vibrational tool for spiritual transformation represent an advanced avenue of exploration. Sound healing, mantra chanting, and specific frequencies harmonize the energetic body and attune it to higher states of consciousness. Advanced practitioners may explore the profound impact of sound on the subtle anatomy, understanding the vibrational resonance as a means of aligning with the cosmic symphony.

A deepening engagement with nature and its spiritual significance becomes a focal point in advanced spiritual practices. The practice of eco-spirituality involves an intellectual understanding of the interconnectedness of all life and a direct communion with the natural world. Advanced seekers may embark on vision quests, undertake extended solitude in the wilderness, or participate in rituals that honor the earth as a sacred living being. Integrating nature-based spirituality invites individuals into a profound relationship with the planetary consciousness.

Exploring the chakras and their energetic dynamics forms an advanced aspect of spiritual practice. While the chakras are introduced in many spiritual traditions, advanced seekers delve into the intricate interplay of these energy centers, seeking to activate, balance, and awaken their full potential. Practices such as chakra meditation, Kundalini yoga, and tantric rituals involve a nuanced understanding of the chakras' influence on physical, emotional, and spiritual well-being.

Exploring the shadow self, rooted in Jungian psychology and embraced in various spiritual traditions, becomes an advanced practice for those committed to self-realization. The shadow represents the unconscious parts of the self, which frequently include suppressed feelings, unfulfilled goals, and unsolved traumas. Advanced seekers engage in shadow work, bringing these hidden aspects into conscious awareness, integrating them, and reclaiming lost parts of the self. This courageous inner journey leads to greater self-acceptance and spiritual wholeness.

The integration of mindfulness into every aspect of daily life becomes an advanced practice in itself. Advanced practitioners cultivate a continuous state of awareness, witnessing the flow of thoughts, emotions, and sensations without attachment. The seamless integration of mindfulness into the fabric of daily existence is a potent tool for self-realization and the embodiment of spiritual wisdom.

In conclusion, exploring advanced spiritual practices is a profound and nuanced journey, requiring dedication, discernment, and a genuine thirst for self-realization. Altered states of consciousness, tantric practices, mystical experiences, esoteric knowledge, psychic development, disciplined sadhana, sacred geometry, sound as a vibrational tool, eco-spirituality, chakra exploration, shadow work, and the seamless integration of mindfulness into daily life represent a rich tapestry of avenues for advanced seekers. These activities are not stand-alone pursuits but interwoven strands that make up a whole spiritual path. As individuals venture into the realms of advanced exploration, may they do so with reverence, humility, and an unwavering commitment to the transformative potential embedded in these sacred practices.

Continuing the journey of self-discovery

The journey of self-discovery is a perpetual odyssey, an ongoing exploration that unfolds across the landscapes of our innermost being. It is an intimate pilgrimage marked by self-reflection, introspection, and a relentless quest to unravel the layers of our identity. As individuals traverse the terrain of their existence, self-discovery becomes a dynamic and evolving process, continually shaped by experiences, relationships, and the ever-unfolding tapestry of life. This section aims to delve into the significance of continuing the journey of self-discovery, exploring the inherent challenges, profound revelations, and the transformative power embedded in the ongoing pursuit of understanding oneself.

At the heart of the journey of self-discovery lies the fundamental question: Who am I? This question is not a mere intellectual inquiry but a contemplative exploration that invites individuals to dive into the depths of their consciousness. The quest for self-understanding goes beyond the surface-level roles, identities, and societal labels, reaching into the essence of one's being. It is peeling away the layers of conditioning, cultural influences, and external expectations to reveal the authentic self that resides beneath.

The journey of self-discovery is often catalyzed by pivotal moments in life—moments of crisis, joy, or profound introspection. Whether prompted by a life-altering event, a period of deep introspection, or an inner longing for meaning, these moments become catalysts for individuals to turn inward and inquire into the nature of their existence. The recognition that life is a continuous journey of growth and self-exploration propels individuals to embark on a path of self-discovery, where each step becomes an opportunity for deeper understanding and self-realization.

One of the profound challenges encountered in the journey of self-discovery is the confrontation with the shadow self. The shadow, a concept rooted in Jungian psychology, represents the aspects of the self that are hidden, repressed, or denied. Delving into the shadow requires a courageous exploration of one's fears, insecurities, and unresolved wounds. It is acknowledging and integrating these aspects rather than rejecting or suppressing them. The journey of self-discovery invites individuals to face the shadows with compassion, recognizing that genuine self-understanding involves embracing the entirety of one's being.

Relationships with oneself and others play a pivotal role in the ongoing journey of self-discovery. Interactions with others are mirrors, reflecting aspects of ourselves that may remain hidden in the solitude of introspection. The dynamics of relationships offer opportunities for self-reflection, revealing patterns, triggers, and growth areas. Whether through the joy of connection, the challenges of conflict, or the wisdom gained from shared experiences, relationships become a fertile ground for self-discovery and a mirror reflecting the multifaceted nature of the self.

The journey of self-discovery extends beyond personal relationships to the broader context of societal and cultural influences. Society often imposes predefined roles, expectations, and norms that shape individual identities. As individuals navigate the currents of societal expectations, self-discovery involves questioning and deconstructing these external influences. It is a process of discerning which aspects of identity are authentically chosen and which are inherited or imposed. The liberation from societal conditioning becomes a profound step toward self-realization.

Cultivating self-awareness is a cornerstone of the ongoing journey of self-discovery. Self-awareness involves observing one's thoughts, emotions, and actions without judgment. People in this condition of conscious presence can perceive and traverse the complexity of their inner landscape with clarity. Reflective journaling, mindfulness, and meditation become instruments for cultivating ongoing mindful living and expanding self-awareness. The journey of self-discovery is intertwined with exploring personal values, beliefs, and life purpose. As individuals grow and evolve, their values and beliefs may transform. Aligning one's life with authentic values and a sense of purpose becomes an ongoing refinement process. The quest for meaning and purpose propels individuals to reassess priorities, make conscious choices, and align their actions with the deeper currents of their authentic selves.

Integrating self-compassion into the journey of self-discovery is vital to navigating the inevitable challenges and setbacks. Self-compassion involves extending the same kindness, understanding, and forgiveness to oneself that one would offer to a dear friend. Embracing imperfections, learning from mistakes, and acknowledging the inherent humanity within oneself become essential components of the ongoing journey. Self-compassion is a nurturing force, fostering resilience and a sense of inner strength as individuals navigate the complexities of self-discovery.

The process of self-discovery is not a linear trajectory but a spiral of continuous growth and expansion. Life unfolds in cycles, providing new insights, challenges, and opportunities for self-reflection. The journey is not about reaching a fixed destination but embracing growth and transformation's fluidity. As individuals navigate the cyclical nature of the trip, they gain a deeper understanding of the ever-changing dynamics of their inner world.

Creativity becomes an avenue for self-expression and exploration in the ongoing journey of self-discovery. Whether through artistic endeavors, writing, or other creative pursuits, individuals find unique ways to give voice to their innermost thoughts, emotions, and experiences. Creativity becomes a mirror reflecting the depths of the unconscious, allowing individuals to explore and express aspects of the self that may elude verbal articulation. Engaging in creative practices becomes a joyful and liberating aspect of the ongoing journey.

The journey of self-discovery often leads individuals to explore their spirituality and the nature of their connection to a higher source or universal consciousness. Spirituality becomes a profoundly personal exploration, encompassing diverse practices such as prayer, meditation, or communing with nature. The search for spiritual understanding provides individuals with a broader context for their existence, offering solace, meaning, and a sense of interconnectedness with something more significant than the individual self.

Integrating mindfulness into daily life becomes a foundational aspect of the ongoing journey of self-discovery. Practicing mindful eating, walking, listening, and engaging with the present moment becomes a transformative way of being. Integrating mindfulness fosters continual awareness, allowing individuals to approach each moment with presence, intention, and a heightened sense of aliveness.

The journey of self-discovery invites individuals to embrace the paradoxes and contradictions within themselves. It is a recognition that the human experience is multifaceted, encompassing light and shadow, strength and vulnerability, joy and sorrow. Embracing these paradoxes becomes a source of wisdom and a testament to the richness of the human experience. The journey involves transcending the limitations of dualistic thinking and embracing the wholeness of one's being.

In conclusion, continuing the journey of self-discovery is a profound and transformative endeavor, requiring dedication, courage, and a commitment to growth. The ongoing exploration of one's identity, the confrontation with the shadow self, the dynamics of relationships, the liberation from societal conditioning, the cultivation of self-awareness, the alignment with personal values and purpose, the integration of self-compassion, the recognition of life's cyclical nature, the expression of creativity, the exploration of spirituality, the practice of mindfulness, and the embrace of paradoxes form integral facets of this perpetual odyssey. As individuals navigate the ever-evolving landscape of self-discovery, may they find solace, inspiration, and a deepening connection to the essence of who they are—an infinite and unfolding journey of becoming.

The limitless potential of a fully awakened Kundalini

The concept of Kundalini, deeply rooted in ancient Eastern spiritual traditions, speaks to a latent, transformative energy residing within the human body. Kundalini, a coiled serpent at the base of the spine, is a powerful energy that can initiate profound spiritual progress and higher states of awareness when it awakens. This part dives into the boundless possibilities of a fully awakened Kundalini, examining the journey of transformation it gives, the pinnacles of spiritual enlightenment, and the enormous effects it can have on the human experience, both individually and collectively.

The awakening of Kundalini is often likened to the uncoiling of a serpent, ascending through the subtle energy channels known as nadis and ultimately reaching the crown of the head, the Sahasrara chakra. This process is not merely symbolic but is believed to shift one's perception, cognition, and awareness radically. A fully awakened Kundalini is thought to bestow heightened states of consciousness, transcending the limitations of ordinary perception and opening the doors to expanded dimensions of reality.

The journey of Kundalini awakening is both a gradual and profound process. As the dormant energy begins to stir, individuals may experience a range of sensations, from subtle energy currents to intense waves of heat or bliss. The activation of the chakras, the energetic centers along the spine, corresponds to the unfolding of specific qualities and capacities within the individual. For instance, awakening the heart chakra may lead to an enhanced capacity for love, compassion, and connection. At the same time, activating the third eye may bring about heightened intuition and insight.

As Kundalini ascends through the chakras, it acts as a purifying and illuminating force, dissolving blockages and energetic knots that may have accumulated over time. This physical purification process extends to mental, emotional, and spiritual dimensions. The release of stagnant energy and the dissolution of old patterns make space for the emergence of a more authentic and integrated self.

A fully awakened Kundalini is said to lead to a state of Samadhi, the pinnacle of meditative absorption and union with the divine. Samadhi is characterized by a profound sense of oneness, where the boundaries between the self and the external world dissolve. In this state, individuals may experience a direct communion with the transcendent, a sense of unity with all of existence, and a dissolution of the egoic self. The awakening of Kundalini is considered a vehicle for transcending the limitations of the individual ego and realizing one's essential nature as a boundless, interconnected being.

The expanded states of consciousness associated with a fully awakened Kundalini extend beyond the confines of ordinary perception. Individuals may report experiences of cosmic consciousness, where they feel intimately connected to the vastness of the cosmos. Time and space may lose their conventional significance, and a sense of eternity and infinity may permeate the awareness. Such experiences are not merely subjective phenomena but are considered intrinsic aspects of the heightened states of consciousness facilitated by the awakened Kundalini.

The limitless potential of a fully awakened Kundalini is intricately tied to enlightenment or self-realization. In various spiritual traditions, enlightenment is viewed as the ultimate goal of human existence—realizing one's true nature and recognizing the interconnectedness of all life. A fully awakened Kundalini catalyzes this profound shift in consciousness, leading individuals to inner illumination, wisdom, and liberation from the cycle of birth and death.

The transformative power of Kundalini is not confined to individual spiritual growth but extends to the collective evolution of humanity. The interconnected nature of all beings implies that the awakening of Kundalini in one individual can contribute to the collective consciousness. As more individuals undergo the transformative journey of Kundalini awakening, the potential for a shift in global consciousness and a more harmonious, compassionate world becomes a tangible possibility. The awakened Kundalini is envisioned as a force that can dissolve the divisive boundaries that separate individuals and foster a sense of unity and interconnectedness on a planetary scale.

However, the limitless potential of a fully awakened Kundalini is accompanied by challenges and potential pitfalls. The intensity of the Kundalini awakening process can give rise to physical, emotional, and psychological disturbances, commonly called the "Kundalini syndrome." These disturbances may include sensations of heat, involuntary movements, emotional upheavals, and altered states of consciousness. It is emphasized in various spiritual traditions that the direction of a knowledgeable mentor or instructor is crucial to navigating the complexities of the Kundalini awakening safely.

The proper preparation for Kundalini awakening involves a foundation of spiritual practices, ethical living, and a genuine commitment to self-realization. Yogic traditions, particularly those that incorporate Kundalini yoga, provide systematic methodologies for preparing the body, mind, and spirit for awakening. Integrating breathwork (pranayama), physical postures (asanas), mantra chanting, and meditation is a holistic approach to preparing the individual for the transformative journey ahead.

The concept of Kundalini is not limited to any particular religious or spiritual tradition. It is a universal archetype found in various forms across cultures, symbolizing the dormant potential for spiritual awakening within each individual. The serpent imagery, present in the caduceus of Hermes in ancient Greek mythology, the Uraeus serpent in Egyptian symbology, and the Kundalini serpent in Hinduism, points to the archetypal nature of this transformative energy. The universal recognition of Kundalini underscores its potential to bridge cultural and religious divides, offering a shared framework for understanding the latent spiritual power within humanity.

In conclusion, the limitless potential of a fully awakened Kundalini is a profound and multifaceted journey, encompassing the expansion of consciousness, the dissolution of egoic boundaries, and the realization of one's essential nature. As individuals embark on the transformative process of Kundalini awakening, they tap into a force that transcends the individual self, contributing to the collective evolution of human consciousness. The challenges and pitfalls associated with Kundalini's awakening underscore the importance of proper preparation and guidance. The archetypal nature of Kundalini highlights its universal relevance, offering a shared understanding of the transformative potential inherent in the human experience. Ultimately, the awakening of Kundalini is an invitation to explore the boundless realms of consciousness, embrace the interconnected nature of existence, and participate in the ongoing evolution of individual and collective consciousness

CONCLUSION

In conclusion, "Rising Serpent: A Guide to Kundalini Awakening - Unlocking Inner Power and Spiritual Transformation" is a comprehensive and insightful companion to the profound journey of Kundalini Awakening. This book, crafted with care and expertise, explores the dormant spiritual energy within, guiding readers through the intricacies of the awakening process. From the foundational understanding of Kundalini to practical techniques for unlocking its transformative power, the e-book offers a roadmap for seekers on the path of spiritual evolution.

Through a carefully structured chapter-based format, the e-book covers many topics, including the roots and principles of Kundalini, practical exercises, and the potential challenges associated with this transformative journey. Each chapter contributes to a holistic understanding of Kundalini, emphasizing its spiritual dimensions and impact on physical, emotional, and mental well-being.

The narrative intertwines ancient wisdom, modern insights, and practical guidance, making Kundalini's complex subject accessible to readers at various stages of their spiritual journey. Whether one is a novice seeking an introduction to Kundalini or an experienced practitioner aiming for a deeper understanding, this e-book acknowledges and values every reader's unique journey, providing valuable insights and tools for unlocking inner power and facilitating spiritual transformation.

The e-book empowers readers to embark on their transformative journey with confidence and awareness by demystifying the concept of Kundalini and offering practical advice. It emphasizes the importance of preparation, ethical living, and the guidance of experienced mentors to navigate the challenges and pitfalls associated with Kundalini awakening.

As readers immerse themselves in the pages of "Rising Serpent," they are equipped with knowledge and inspired to embrace the limitless potential within. The e-book stands as a beacon for those yearning for spiritual growth, inviting them to embark on self-discovery, inner power, and profound spiritual transformation. With its insightful guidance and accessible approach, "Rising Serpent" is a valuable resource for anyone seeking to unlock the dormant energy within and traverse the transformative path of Kundalini's awakening.

Thank you for buying and reading/ listening to our book. If you found this book useful/ helpful please take a few minutes and leave a review on the platform where you purchased our book. Your feedback matters greatly to us.

www.ingramcontent.com/pod-product-compliance
Lightning Source LLC
LaVergne TN
LVHW010343070526
838199LV00065B/5776